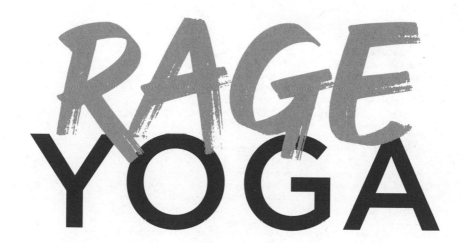

RAGE YOGA

UNLEASH YOUR INNER BADASS

LINDSAY ISTACE

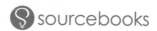
sourcebooks

Copyright © 2021 by Lindsay Istace
Cover and internal design © 2021 by Sourcebooks
Cover design by Heather VenHuizen/Sourcebooks
Cover images © David McKenzie/DMacStudios, phochi/Getty Images
Internal illustrations by Chrissy Lau
Internal images © Ani_Ka/Getty Images, Anna Tkachenko/Getty Images, irinabogomolova/Getty Images, non-exclusive/Getty Images, Popova Anna/Getty Images, vectorplusb/Getty Images, Freepik

Sourcebooks and the colophon are registered trademarks of Sourcebooks.

Published by Sourcebooks
P.O. Box 4410, Naperville, Illinois 60567-4410
(630) 961-3900
sourcebooks.com

Library of Congress Cataloging-in-Publication Data

Names: Istace, Lindsay, author.
Title: Rage yoga : release your inner badass / Lindsay Istace.
Description: Naperville, Illinois : Sourcebooks, [2021]
Identifiers: LCCN 2021001202 |
Subjects: LCSH: Hatha yoga--Popular works. | Exercise--Popular works. |
    Self-care, Health--Popular works.
Classification: LCC RA781.7 .I88 2021 | DDC 613.7/046--dc23
LC record available at https://lccn.loc.gov/2021001202

Printed and bound in the United States of America.
VP 10 9 8 7 6 5 4 3 2 1

Yo, Uncle Bob! You're one of the most unconventional and important influences I have had in my life. You encouraged my love of art and adventure. You taught me to consider seemingly impossible possibilities. You've given me a strong heart, foul mouth, and an appreciation for questionable haircuts. Thanks, jerk. I love you.

CONTENTS

WHAT IS RAGE YOGA?

Before you read any further, I want to take a moment to answer some of the most common questions that I get asked about Rage Yoga.

What the Actual Fuck Is Rage Yoga?

Rage Yoga is an alternative approach to yoga's traditional practices and teachings and to those we find in conventional Western studios. It's not about giving tradition the middle finger, despite whatever you may have read online. It's not about holding on to anger for the sake of screaming while you stretch either. It's about learning how to accept your uncomfortable emotions, dismantle them, and even use them constructively to lead a life that is Zen as fuck. Rage Yoga can be an attitude, a lifestyle, and a method of unleashing your most *Badass Self*. You don't have to be angry to practice Rage Yoga, but if you are, you definitely don't need to hide it here. We get messy, we get loud, and we're not afraid of the darkness inside us. Rage Yoga is for the weirdos, anarchists, and unapologetic badasses of the yoga world.

Why Do People Practice Rage Yoga?

Rage Yoga tends to bring people to the mat who otherwise might not step into the yoga world. Despite being curious or knowing that it could have massive benefits for them, these people tend to shy away from yoga because they find conventional practices intimidating or because they feel that they need to be something or someone else in order to fit in.

Take Owen, for example. "I'm a forty-year-old metalhead. I don't exactly fit in at a traditional yoga studio. Rage Yoga gives me the opportunity to do a practice in a comfortable, welcoming environment." Owen says that his instructor, Carri, introduced him to Rage Yoga and showed him yoga in a new light that made sense to him.

There are tons of others who don't feel like they fit into the typical yoga scene, but in a Rage Yoga class, they can feel at home. They know they will not be judged based on their skill level or their knowledge—or lack thereof—of yoga. Let's get real for a second. When you first start a yoga program, you don't feel Zen and relaxed. You feel frustrated because all the poses are new, you don't know the terminology, you don't know proper breathing techniques, and your body does not move the way you want it to. You might feel like a bumbling baby giraffe just trying to play it cool and draw as little attention to yourself as possible.

Rage Yoga leans in to that discomfort and gives you permission to feel that frustration...as well as all the frustration of other Bullshit that we tend to collect and carry around like emotional hoarders. Then it creates a safe environment to release all that Bullshit and move past your inner critic. It encourages you to be authentic in your practice and in yourself, even if it isn't perfect or pretty. It opens up accessibility to yoga, removes barriers to entry, and helps you find your voice and stop censoring yourself. Here, it's okay to scream at the top of your lungs. It's okay to let that F bomb out and throw down a middle finger (which I prefer to call a "fist unicorn"). By empowering yourself to release whatever you're holding on to (often through anger, laughter, or tears), you will find you feel less alone and you're more readily able to connect to others as well as yourself.

Whether you're looking for an accessible door into the world of yoga or an alternative practice to add to your own, this just might be the practice you're looking for. Welcome to the self-loving—and cathartic as fuck—world of Rage Yoga.

It's certainly not for everyone, and that is okay. In fact...

Fuck ass!

BLOODY BASTARD!
DAMN MOTHERFUCKER!
FUCKING SHITTY FART FACE!

I forgot to mention that we also love foul language…and puns. *You've been warned.*

I just figured we'd filter some people out right from the start and save everyone some time. Are you still there? Great!

How Did Rage Yoga Become a Thing?

Long story short: Rage Yoga was born in a dingy-ass basement apartment in Alberta, Canada, in 2015, during one of the coldest and most depressing winters of my life.

I've had a very strong physical practice my entire life, even before I called it yoga. As a kid, I was typically found stretching, dancing, and balancing everywhere on everything. I also had a very strong curiosity about the potential of the mind and the nature of the universe. I thought a lot about spirituality, the soul, the origin of time, the human experience, the meaning of life… All of it was fascinating to me! When I paired my movement practice, or play, with this deeper mode of thinking, I found my happy place, and I retreated there often without realizing the meditative value of it.

I wasn't some super-enlightened kid who had it all sorted out from the beginning. Fuck no! I'm still figuring it out every day. I was just fortunate to have a natural interest in this deeper personal world, because as a rather unstable kid with an absent support system, it was the one healthy coping mechanism I had! It gave me the strength to get through my shittiest times and the insight to learn how to do better. Although the depth and characteristics of that mind-body happy place continue to change and

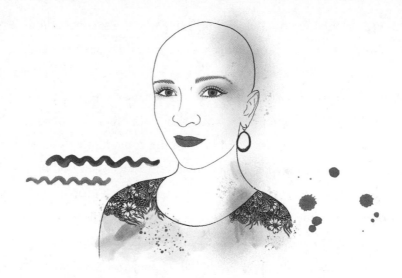

develop through the years, it has been one of my few stable pillars in life. It gives me a sense of connection to something beyond my individual experience. It keeps me happy and sane (enough). It is an important and invaluable part of my life.

So I guess that's why it makes sense that I essentially ran away to join the circus. The meditative aspect of the movement and the process of learning difficult, new skills satisfied my need for that mind-body happy place. I started with crystal ball juggling (a.k.a. contact juggling) and then fire dancing. Then I decided to become a contortionist. Unbeknownst to me at the time, however, one does not simply become a contortionist. It is not that easy! At twenty-two, I went to Beijing to study contortion under badass coaches, unaware of the intensely educational hell I was about to put myself through. If I had known at the time how physically and mentally excruciating it would be, I probably woulda nope'd right the fuck out.

Although in the long run it ended up being one the smartest things I have ever done, taking on this challenge was an entirely foolish pursuit.

The Chinese students thought I was nuts because I was choosing to enter into the grueling world of traditional circus arts. Few of them actually wanted to be there. They were kids who hadn't met the incredibly high academic standards necessary to excel in the conventional school system. In an environment in which most of their adult success would be based on the achievements they made in their youth, this was a problem. Their families often didn't have a lot of money, so in the end, these parents made the safest gamble they could think of to procure a promising future for their children—and it was circus arts. These kids may not have had the intellectual genius needed to make it to the top of conventional classes, but they were fit and physically capable kids. At the school, they would be molded into circus machines. They lived on campus and only got to go home on special occasions. Some of them seemed to like it, but most just accepted it begrudgingly because they didn't have much say in the matter. Then there was me, the strange foreigner who had flown halfway across the world and paid a lot of money to willingly subject myself to this intense training.

There is a saying in the circus community: "Circus is pain." They're not fucking around. Sometimes my teacher would hold my legs and make me stay in handstands for such long periods of time that I thought my body would collapse in on itself or that my wrists would explode. When my calves got sore and tight, she would get me to lie on my stomach. Then she would use her feet, walking on my calves, to massage the muscles using her body weight. I was instructed to hold stretches for absurd amounts of time, sometimes with heavy weights on my body to make the stretch even deeper. It was intense! But the toughest part of class was when we had to stretch our splits.

Every day, when it came time for splits, we'd line up to wait our turn. I often found myself waiting in line and wondering why the hell I was doing this voluntarily. It felt as if a cow willingly got in line at a slaughterhouse! On my turn, I would lie on my back with a teacher on each leg. For front splits, one teacher would sit on my lower leg to pin it to the ground. The other teacher would forcefully hoist my second leg up to my face. They would hold it there and count to forty, pushing deeper as the time passed. Then they would angle the lifted leg slightly across my body and count all over again. This was followed by middle splits. I would stay on my back while the teachers took my legs wide and aggressively forced them into the ground. Then, once again, they would count to forty.

A funny thing happens when you're put into extreme situations like this—time seems to slow right down. I could hear my teacher counting, but it seemed like her lips were moving even slower than Keanu Reeves dodging bullets in *The Matrix*. It became easy to get caught up and lose myself in the intensity of it. My body wanted to panic, lose control of my breath, and tense up in defense. This is the body's natural survival response to this type of stress. But there was no point in fighting it. The teachers didn't care if I fought, protested, or cried. The teacher was going to hold me there, even if it was agonizing torture, and they were going to count to forty. I could either hate it, spending every second of what felt like eternity regretting my very existence and every choice I'd ever made, or I could relax.

Relaxing into extreme discomfort is difficult, but it is a skill you can learn. You keep your breath steady, and in the middle of the hell that is your current experience, you find a spot of calm. In a way, you surrender to it and befriend the terrible sensation. This makes it significantly less terrible, and instead of breaking you down, it makes you stronger, both physically and mentally. It's much harder to do this instead of panicking and freaking out! But in the end, it's less painful, you're less likely to injure yourself, and you see progress a lot faster. You also spend less energy making yourself miserable!

To get through classes, I needed to have a lot of this mental and physical discipline. The training really took a toll on me. Tears of pain and/or frustration were not an uncommon sight. It wasn't a relaxing practice; it was incredibly agonizing work! Still, rain or shine, good or bad day, I would show up for my classes and do the work.

Another difficult aspect of my time at the school was the language barrier. The vast majority of the people around me didn't speak my language, and although I tried really fucking hard, I couldn't speak any Mandarin. Eventually I learned how to say "pain," "no pain," "beer," and "thank you." I also, for obvious reasons, learned to count to forty, but that wasn't going to help me make real connections with people! Until conversation wasn't an option, I hadn't realized how much I distracted myself with other people to avoid my inner world or how heavily I relied on humor to relate without feeling vulnerable. Although there were a couple of English-speaking foreign students, the people around me seemed unreachable. I felt very alone. I had nothing to distract myself from the storm I had inside me, yet I had to turn inside to get through the physical pain of my classes. So I turned inside, looked at that storm, and took it head-on. I found my Badass Self.

I'm a big fan of do-nothing days. If every day could include some yoga, Netflix bingeing, a beer, and a nap, that would just be de-fucking-lightful!

However, this wouldn't actually be much benefit in the long run. The truth is that it's the hard days that force us to grow. To overcome struggle, we often have to dig and connect to something deeper inside ourselves. It can take some work to wake it up, but we all have a higher level of being inside us. God, spirit, higher self, the universe...call it Harold for all I care! I prefer to call it my Badass Self. This deeper thing, whatever name you give it, is resilient as fuck. It is strong, confident, and wise. It is a space of calm and stillness, even in the face of chaos and change. My training in Beijing wasn't fun, but it was one of the most impactful times of my life because it forced me to go to that deeper place.

Tapping into my Badass Self helped me get through my training in one piece and enjoy it, even when it was hard. It also gave me what I needed to face the mess of my inner world. Now that I had opened that door, a lot of my darkness was bubbling to the forefront. It was a mosaic of traumas, insecurities, broken coping mechanisms, and moldy emotional baggage. My Badass Self allowed me to see these things, spot my own weaknesses, and find the strength to face them. That meditative state of befriending pain that I had honed in my physical training began to transfer over into what became an introspective practice. I wanted to do better, not just in my flexibility goals but as a person. I started to broaden my practice, venturing into the worlds of philosophy and religious study. I explored different methods of developing a mind-body connection through meditation techniques and movement. I fell in love with learning, and at this point, my personal practice truly started becoming yogic in nature.

Because of this, I started to recognize the cracks in my own life. I wasn't attached to the idea of attaining personal perfection, but I was committed to, at the very least, being less shitty. This change caused me to look long and hard at the things I used as crutches and the many ways self-sabotage popped up in my life. I began to examine myself, keeping a keen eye open, watching for toxic influences, and calling myself out on my own Bullshit. Still, when you decide to make this kind of change, there are two different battlefields. There is the one in your mind, and then there is the one all around you. I worked hard to change the landscape of my internal world, but that was only getting me so far. When I started looking at the life I had created for myself, I found that my metaphorical garden desperately needed some weeding. This was when I realized that I needed to break up with my partner.

This wasn't a decision I came to happily. It was my first real long-term adult relationship, and I had a ring on my finger. When we got together, this partner had been the person I needed. He had challenged me to grow and to pursue my goals. Without him, I would have missed out on many experiences and friendships that have greatly impacted and shaped my life. I'm eternally grateful to have had that relationship; it's an important chapter of my life! Yet when I looked at it truthfully, it was unhealthy. The passionate relationship that had once made us both happy and encouraged us to grow had deteriorated into codependent enabling. We had gotten stuck, plateauing in booze and depressive isolation. Now I had changed in ways that made him incapable of being the person I needed in my new chapter. In turn, this new me was incapable of being the partner he needed without faking it like a poorly cast actor in a shitty play. It had to end.

No matter what anyone says, being the one to end a relationship doesn't make it any easier. He really did love me, and I felt like I betrayed him. I felt the guilt of being the one who burned an entire future to the ground. No matter the circumstances, breakups are fucking painful; they come with hurt, confusion, even fear, and all these things are valid. These hard emotions can crush a person, but you can use the broken pieces to make something new. Little did I know that those were the broken pieces that would end up creating Rage Yoga.

There's no nice way to say it—it fucked me up! I did my best to keep myself together, but I was a whirlwind of strong and chaotic emotions, and without a healthy way to work through what I was feeling, I ended up falling apart. We've all been there, right? Eating ice cream for breakfast with a glass of boxed wine, spending days at a time in the same pajamas, and staring blankly at walls while trying to process the white noise in the back of your brain. Yeah. It was one of those. This phase was certainly a cathartic distraction, and maybe, for a short while, that was helpful! After a month, however, it became a little excessive. I knew I needed to stop being a gremlin and get back to feeling like a person again. I picked myself up, took a much-needed shower, and (finally) put on some clean clothes.

Then I got my ass out the door and took it to a yoga class.

Just because I was ready to leave my apartment doesn't mean I was suddenly okay. I was *not* okay. I tried to keep it quiet, but I was still fighting off tears in resting poses, and sometimes an angry groan or sad sigh would escape me in deeper postures. People didn't seem to like that. I got a lot of funny looks and was treated the way most people treat rashes...like maybe if they ignored me long enough, I would just go away! Even more so than just being in general public, it felt like the yoga studio was a place where you needed to pretend to have your shit together. But I couldn't fake it; my shit was scattered as fuck. I felt like an outcast who had spoiled the immaculate and serene atmosphere of the studio. My attempts to make my pain palatable enough for other people weren't fooling anyone or helping me. So I took my ass home again.

Away from the awkward pressures that I felt in a conventional studio, something magical happened. While I was alone in that dingy-ass basement apartment, I found what I needed.

By the way, if your mind just got dirty there, then you are wrong…

…but I like the way you think.

If you search #yoga on any social media platform, you're going to find a wealth of beautiful photos. There will be stunning people in flawless outfits, doing yoga postures in Pinterest-perfect spaces. The caption is often a motivational quote, and it's rare that these people wrote it themselves. You know what I'm talking about, right? Yeah? Well, this was exactly the opposite of that.

I was sobbing in hip openers, letting out battle cries in my warrior poses, and laughing maniacally in forward bends. I'm sure my neighbors thought I was clinically insane, but who cares! Growing isn't pretty; in fact, it can get downright messy. My mat became a safe space to let out what I had been holding in, and it turned out that it was a hell of a lot more than just a breakup! It was a lifetime's worth of built-up anxieties, hurt, anger, trauma, and fear that had been swept out of sight. Even if I screamed or ugly cried, by the end of the session, I'd feel lighter and stronger. I began to stop wallowing and became strong enough to let go and then vulnerable enough to rise above it. It. Felt. Fantastic.

To process and overcome our uncomfortable emotions, trauma,

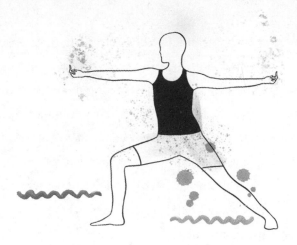

or general Bullshit, we need to acknowledge them. We can't just tuck all that into the back of the closet, pretend everything is okay, and smile like nothing is wrong until everyone (hopefully ourselves included) believes it. Although we all wish it were the case, these things don't just disappear if we stop paying attention to them. That shit just stays hidden away for a while, where it mutates and comes back out later to smack us upside the face with mutant strength! You best believe that a mutant-strength upside-the-face smacking is going to fuck your day up a hell of a lot harder than a regular smack upside the face.

I wanted to find a community where I could keep doing this kind of practice. I wanted to be able to share the things about me that weren't pretty or perfectly serene and centered. I wanted to see what a yoga practice could look like if people left their filters at the door and didn't sugarcoat their feelings. I knew now that there was a lot of power in embracing, maybe even befriending, your own messiness, and I wanted to share that with others! I couldn't find an existing community that fit what I was looking for, so I decided to try to make one myself.

What began as an at-home practice became an alternative workshop at a festival, which led to another workshop. Soon, that lead to weekly sessions at Dickens, a community-minded basement pub and kick-ass music venue in Calgary, Alberta. In the beginning, our community was small (although *very* enthusiastic), and I thought it would stay that way. I had no idea how many people would want what Rage Yoga offered.

It didn't take long for the word to get out. A local paper wrote about us after a couple of months of weekly classes, and then, a couple of days later, the local television news featured us.

Cool, I thought. *Maybe we'll get a couple extra people out to Dickens next week!*

HA!

News stations in the United States picked up the story, and suddenly everyone was talking about Rage Yoga, even Kelly Ripa on *Live with Kelly and Michael*! Everything blew up, seemingly overnight, and I was doing radio interviews for stations in New York, New Zealand, Australia, Russia, and throughout North America. Every day, I was waking up to a bloated email inbox full of franchise offers, requests for classes all around the world, and even requests for mentorship. Many people wrote me out of gratitude, and some even took the time to write hate mail. (*I fucking LOVE hate mail!*) I had a never-ending stream of messages on Facebook from friends, family, and strangers. They were sharing news articles, asking questions, and telling me how even their hairdresser was talking about it. Throughout this crazy roller coaster, one thing was clear: I was not alone.

At this point, Rage Yoga was bigger than just me. There was a small group of amazing people around me who helped run the classes and plan for what the future might hold. They also helped keep me sane in the process! We built a solid community around our local classes, but the demand was bigger than what we could offer from the back room at Dickens. Around the world, people wanted Rage Yoga. So we kept growing.

Since then, we've shared Rage Yoga with people all over. We've organized retreats, my favorite being the one in Glasgow (which is now the place I want to haunt when I die). We've done a cross-country tour doing workshops and created many different online classes to reach those who want to practice at home. Eventually, the demand for more in-person classes got so big that we created the Rage Yoga Certified Badass Instructor Program! I'm proud of our incredible teachers, many of whom teach regularly in their local communities or have created online video programs. And now...oh, look! A Rage Yoga book!

Yoga's traditional roots are in Indian religion, which has many different breath practices, forms of meditation, and schools of philosophy. In the Western world, we don't really know how to categorize yoga. People often label it as either fitness, self-help, or spirituality. In essence, it is a little bit of all of these, and Rage Yoga is no exception! In this book, you will find loads of traditional poses, practices, and philosophies. You'll find lots of Rage-style additions and twists too.

We're getting physical, philosophical, and sometimes even a bit self-help-y, but if you think that means this book is going to blow smoke up your ass, then you're sorely mistaken! I'm not going to tell you that you're made of stardust or shove spirituality down your throat. I'm here to help you become Zen as fuck and unleash your most Badass Self.

So if you're ready, can I get a "Fuck yeah!"?

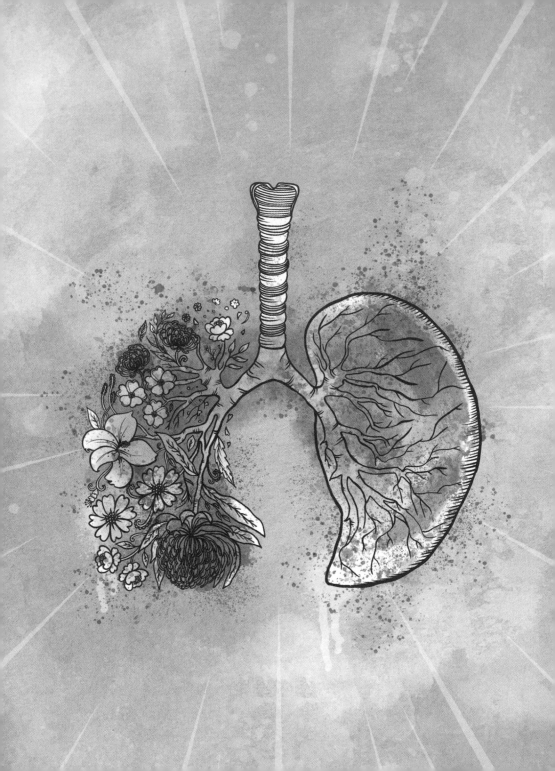

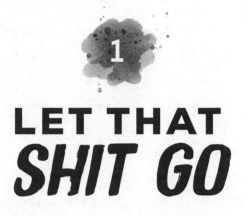

LET THAT
SHIT GO

**"A journey of a thousand miles
begins with a single step."**
−LAO TZU

No matter how outrageous or awe-inspiring, every journey begins the same way. Eventually, each journey grows in its own direction, developing chapters and characteristics unique to itself, but in their infancy, they all look the same. They start out small and simple. They begin with a single step.

We often forget this when we start looking around at what everyone else seems to be doing. Although sometimes it might be inspiring, the success stories of others can be really intimidating, especially when we see them online! Social media is full of success stories, curated by those who share them. People frequently leave out the awkward first steps of their journey and jump straight to the end, where there are pretty pictures and polished results. It's easy to fall into the trap of thinking, "They can do all these things because they're special, and I can't because I'm not." But that's bullshit. For example, Lady Gaga wasn't just suddenly Lady Gaga. Sure, she was "born this way," but to grow into herself and accomplish the things she has accomplished, she went on a journey. This is true of anyone who has ever done anything worth talking about! I promise that all those journeys started out small and simple. They began with a single step.

Unless your plan is to run an actual marathon or something, then try not to take this too literally. A step isn't just the simple moving forward of a foot. This step consists of two parts, one part direction and one part momentum.

For the journey that you're about to embark on through this book, the direction is obvious. It's in the freakin' title! If you thought this book would guide you toward being a master mechanic or culinary genius, then you're shit out of luck. We're headed for the land of unfuckwithable badasses. We're becoming Zen as fuck. That is our direction. Now all we need is a little momentum to get us started.

This is where your epic journey begins. **Right. Here.**

It begins with a *breath*.

There's a good chance that right now, you're staring at this page like you've just smelled a fart, like *"Say whaaaat?!"*

It's anticlimactic, I know. Here I am, just casually dropping words like *epic*, and the big reveal is breathing. But hey, I did say that all epic journeys start out small and simple, and I meant it! No, it's not as grand as a popular #yoga photo on social media or as flashy as an inspirational quote scrawled across your yoga mat in a loopy font, yet breath is the cornerstone of a yoga practice. Breath will be the mother of momentum on your journey. It will be the wind in your sails, the deciding factor in where you can go and how quickly you get there.

You might be thinking, "It's not that hard. I've been breathing since I was born. I'm breathing right now, dammit!"

It's true! Assuming you were a healthy baby, when you were born, you knew how to breathe. It was a natural rhythm, your personal metronome. You breathed deep into your belly and used your lungs to their full capacity. You did all this without a thought and without an instruction manual. But eventually, this all changed.

Shallow Breathing

Perhaps this is because of how complicated things seem to get as we get older. Suddenly, we have social responsibilities and need to find our own way to make a living. There are countless decisions we must make every day that affect our lives and the lives of the people around us. There is no shortage of opportunities to get caught up in stress and anxiety! Just in case the mental overload wasn't enough to make it difficult to breathe, our societal script also says we should have flat stomachs. This causes a lot of people to retrain themselves, consciously or subconsciously, to take shallow breaths into their chests and to avoid letting their stomachs expand.

Everyone develops unhealthy breathing patterns at some point in their lives. Well, maybe I shouldn't say "everyone." I'm sure those who were raised in an ashram or monastery with daily breath exercises didn't, but

I'm going to go out on a limb and say that doesn't apply to you. For whatever reasons, internal or external, we end up adopting shallow breathing. This becomes an irregular rhythm, our own personal broken metronome. We take short breaths and barely use our lungs to their full capacity. We do this all without realizing how inefficient and awkward it is. It's a hell of a lot more than just awkward though. It has a huge negative impact on our mental and physical health!

Shallow breathing creates a stress response in our bodies, which can then turn into panic attacks, dry mouth, and fatigue. Even worse than just creating a stress response, shallow breathing can actually reinforce *stress as a habit* in our bodies. That means that in the same way a person can develop a habit of cracking their knuckles all the time or saying "like" every two seconds, the body makes a habit of being stressed out. This can wreak havoc on the body's immune system, leaving the body susceptible to disease and possibly aggravating preexisting medical conditions. It can also mess with sleep cycles, cause further fatigue, and raise blood pressure.

Shallow breathing can even create problems for our muscles. This is because shallow breathing bypasses the stomach and brings the breath into the chest, which uses different muscles to expand the lungs. Instead of using the muscles that are meant to help us breathe, we end up relying on different muscles in the chest, neck, and shoulders. It's like bringing your car to your local barista for an oil change instead of going to a mechanic. These muscles *can* get the job done, but they're not great at it. The extra workload can make the muscles tired and tense, often resulting in pain and headaches. This can eventually affect the body's posture, which can lead to yet another world of problems.

Shallow breathing can cause a lot of issues, you see, and the opposite is also true. Many different health conditions, like asthma, blood clots, or physical injury, can cause shallow breathing. It can be a bit of a chicken-or-egg scenario, and it may not be clear exactly which came first. One thing is sure though: we've all got ninety-nine problems, but shallow breathing doesn't chronically *have* to be one!

But what exactly does a healthy breath look like?

CYCLICAL BREATH EXERCISE

The cyclical breath is made up of three parts that all work together to make one super badass whole-body breath. The three parts include your stomach, ribs, and chest. Before you can get a cyclical breath going, you gotta get a solid feel for all these parts individually. Before a lasagna becomes lasagna, all the layers are separate. The cheese, sauce, and noodles are individual parts that unite in making a multilayered culinary delight (that I am definitely craving in this moment). Let's get in touch with those breathing layers before we bring them together.

Start by lying on your back and placing your fingertips over your belly. On your inhale, focus on bringing the air into your belly and feeling your fingers rise. On the exhale, feel your fingers lower. During this part of the exercise, focus on bringing your breath into just your stomach.

Once you've got a feel for this, bring your fingertips a little bit higher onto your lower ribs. This time, you want to focus on bringing the air into the ribs only. On the inhale, your fingertips rise, and on the exhale, they lower.

Then—you guessed it—move your fingertips up onto your chest. Rest them just below your clavicle, and repeat the practice of isolating your breath in the one area. Do this one more time, taking a couple of deep breaths into each isolated area, making sure to engage the other two as little as possible as you go.

Before we carry on, can we take a second to talk about this? It's weird, right? It feels really fucked up to only breathe actively into one part of the body, yet it's something we do subconsciously all the time. It feels shitty, and it's bad for your health, so let's cut that crap out, yeah?

Now we're ready to add the layers together, like a breath lasagna. Begin on your back. On your inhale, bring your breath into your stomach. Keep breathing in as you let the breath roll up into your ribs and then into your chest. Follow the same order as you exhale. Let your stomach lower, then your ribs, and finally your chest. Follow this pattern, allowing it to become an awesome wave rolling through you. Repeat this cyclical breath ten times...or more if you just can't get enough!

Prana

Proper breathing optimizes the body and mind. After the cyclical breath exercise, you may notice that you feel different. Perhaps you are more energized, relaxed, or grounded. With this experience, plus the information in this chapter so far and maybe simply using your own common sense, we can all agree that breathing is good, yes? Western science has embraced the fact that the quality of our breathing has a strong effect on our health. There have been many studies done on the topic, and the consensus boils down to the obvious: deep breathing is good for your health. But traditional yogic philosophy takes this further with the concept of prana.

The words *prana* and *breath* are almost synonymous when talking about yogic breath practices, but they are actually two very different things! Breath is...breath! It's air entering and exiting the lungs. Prana is different. Prana is a Sanskrit word that (when boiled down) means "energy of the universe." It's said to be the divine energy given to us by the universe. It's a hell of a lot more than just air entering the body.

Western thinking often says that our conscious experience is made from the body, mind, and senses. Yogic thinking says that all those things are made of prana, the spark and source of life. The mind and senses are just expressions of it that are being experienced through the body, which is also made of prana! In a nutshell: prana is divine, life-giving, good stuff, and breathing is said to be the primary method of absorbing it into the body. Once inside the body, prana gets to work cleansing the body, mind, and spirit. With this cleansing, prana is said to connect us to the divine and make enlightenment possible.

You may choose to view this through a modern science lens, a traditional yogic lens, or even a somewhere-in-between lens! No matter which way you want to look at it, the fact is that the breath holds a lot of power, and relearning how to do it properly is a fucking fabulous idea. Reduced stress and anxiety? Yes please! Improved mood and memory? Sign me up! Increased capacity for concentration and a stronger sense of peace of mind? Fuck yeah! All this is possible by building a healthy breath practice.

Breathing is a habit that is strongly hardwired into us, and relearning it takes time. We can't consciously police every single breath we take, and it won't magically become perfect overnight. Change comes with consistent practice. Ideally, this looks like carving some time out of the day, even just a couple of minutes, to sit down and focus on it. This isn't *Candy Crush* or *Angry Birds* or whatever cell phone game the kids are playing these days! Instant gratification is not a feature of anything long-lasting, so this will take some persistence. That's why they call it a *practice*.

In yoga, the practice of controlling the breath is called *pranayama*. There are many different techniques and types of pranayama. There are also many different uses! Although the absorption of prana is the number one purpose of pranayama, there are specific breath techniques to help accomplish other goals as well, from supercharging energy to calming down, from warming our bodies to cooling them off. Whatever your need is, there is probably a pranayama practice for it. We won't be covering all of them here, but there are plenty of resources out there for your perusing delight.

If you can maintain control over your breath, then you can get through just about anything. It's probably not going to give you superpowers. If an anvil falls on your head, then you're still likely toast. However, people have used breath control to survive terrible things, such as torture. On a less depressing note, they've also used it to achieve mind-melting orgasms! I'm referring, of course, to Tantric sex and not autoerotic asphyxiation. Although people have done that too. I'm not here to kink shame; I'm here to help you get Zen as fuck! So for now, let's supercharge the breath with these two simple instructions:

INHALE THE GOOD SHIT.
EXHALE THE BULLSHIT.

Adding these cues to the breath is like having a colored tint on your sunglasses. It doesn't necessarily change the experience itself, but it does change how you perceive it. The goal of these cues is to nourish your Badass Self by bringing in positive, ass-kicking qualities while letting go of stuff that is not so awesome. Every time you use them, you're making small reinforcements in your mind and setting yourself up for maximum excellence. Let's take a closer look at these cues.

Inhale the Good Shit

The Good Shit can be anything you want: confidence, strength, patience, compassion, joy, forgiveness, etc. Imagine pulling these qualities in with the breath and absorbing them into yourself. The goal here is to bring in whatever qualities you need to find contentment in the present.

I want to note that when I say "contentment in the present," I don't mean to sound like one of those assholes. You know...the ones who say stuff like "just be happy" or "good vibes only" or "you're so pretty when you smile!" It's easy to be content during the highs of life, but during the low parts, it can be significantly harder. Finding contentment in the present doesn't mean being able to magically think things into perfection or brainwashing ourselves to believe they are perfect. We should always strive to make things better, but nothing will ever be completely perfect. There will always be some level of conflict between people, systems will always have flaws, and we will never get everything we want.

During the harder parts, being content in the present keeps us resilient so we don't get overwhelmed or swept under the current of life. It allows us the freedom to enjoy the beauty and find a place to breathe in the middle of it all, even if only for a moment. It lets us be steady in our breath and in ourselves. This way, we can roll up our sleeves and take life by the balls or, at the very least, just feel a little less shitty during a low point.

INHALE THE GOOD SHIT

Find yourself a comfortable position and, if it doesn't feel weird for you, close your eyes. Take a couple of deep natural breaths to settle in and make yourself real cozy. Begin taking your breaths in and out through your nose. Bonus points if you can work in some of the cyclical breaths that we did in the last exercise, letting your breath come and go in waves.

On your next inhale, think about pulling in all the Good Shit. On the following inhale, pull it in and then picture it dissolving into your body. Continue to pull Good Shit into you with every breath, absorbing it and letting it become part of you. Confidence, strength, patience, happiness... Whatever it is you need right now, it is in the air.

Keep.

Breathing.

It.

In.

After at least ten repetitions, check in with your body. Different parts of you may feel varying sensations: warmth, lightness, coldness, tension, etc. Take note of these without trying to change them.

Exhale the Bullshit

The Bullshit is anything that isn't making you better physically, mentally, or emotionally. It could be fear, self-doubt, a memory, disgust, etc. Imagine letting these go with the breath. It's like deleting old videos from your phone to free up space for something better. Why hold on to duplicate images or the photos you accidentally took of your legs when your finger slipped? Free up that space for something better! Perhaps photos of your loved ones, pictures of animals wearing tiny hats, or whatever it is that makes you smile. To make room for more Good Shit, you have to clear out some of the Bullshit.

Everyone has Bullshit; it's a by-product of being alive! Be sure to let it go without demonizing it. Demonizing it is, in a roundabout way, demonizing ourselves. Instead, think about it like jogging with a pebble in your shoe. Being angry at yourself for having a pebble in your shoe is pretty silly. You didn't go out, find a pebble, and then place it in your shoe intentionally. Being mad at the pebble is also pretty silly. It didn't put itself there on purpose, and it's certainly not going to apologize. It's a pebble, dammit! It's inanimate, so it's weird to demonize it. Still, it being there is not helpful to you on your jog. You might need to shake out a bunch of pebbles. Or you might find that the same ones keep getting back in there somehow. That's *not* weird. Just pause for a minute, take off your shoe, remove the pebble, and keep going. Then repeat as necessary.

This is also how you should treat your own Bullshit. It's not as easy as taking something out of your shoe. Sometimes it takes effort, and you may have to let go of it multiple times. But why would you keep holding on to something that only causes you discomfort and slows you down? Instead, *inhale the Good Shit* and *exhale the Bullshit.*

EXHALE THE BULLSHIT

Get comfortable, my fantastic friend. Close your eyes if you like, and take a couple of deep natural breaths to settle into your body. Begin taking your breaths in and out through your nose. Aim to get some cyclical breath going on here, letting it come and go in waves.

On your next exhale, release that Bullshit—any physical or emotional things that are stored up inside you, making you feel bogged down. On your following exhale, expel more of the buildup that has collected over time and is in any way making you feel less than awesome. Keep letting that Bullshit go, telling it kindly to fuck right off so you can make space for new and better things. Whatever that Bullshit is, it's not your obligation to hold on to it.

Keep.

Breathing.

It.

Out.

After at least ten repetitions, check in with your body and notice any new physical sensations. Take note of any differences you might feel in these sensations compared to what you felt after the first exercise.

Feel lighter? Now let's tie it all together!

INHALE THE GOOD SHIT AND EXHALE THE BULLSHIT

Find yourself a comfortable seated position and, if you like, close your eyes. Get settled in with a couple of deep and natural breaths. Begin breathing through your nose, in and out, letting it come and go in waves.

With every inhale, bring in all that fantastic Good Shit. Let it dissolve into you, reinforcing your Badass Self. With every exhale, the stale and stagnant stuff leaves you, carried out with your breath. Every inhale displaces the Bullshit buildup, renews you, and builds you stronger. Every exhale takes more of the unwanted residue away and leaves you lighter. Let this sensation roll through you.

Inhale Good Shit.

Exhale Bullshit.

After at least ten repetitions, check in with your body. Take note of any and all new physical sensations.

How did that feel? Better than chewing tinfoil, right? You can tap into the power of your breath at any time. It's an amazing tool that allows you to be more resilient, more present, and more badass. Best of all, it's available 24/7. Still, for most of us, the breath is an incredibly underrated superpower that we rarely use because we keep forgetting that we have this power in the first place! Remember to use it. It's Good Shit.

Expectation

A common piece of Bullshit that we find ourselves needing to let go of is expectation. Expectation can be a real buzzkill, and it comes in many forms. There are expectations that people place on one another, the ones we place on the world around us, and those we place on ourselves. What expectation really boils down to is having an attachment to a certain outcome.

In theory, being attached to a certain outcome makes sense. We all really just want to be happy, right? Our expectations are tied to that desire, even if the connection isn't obvious. However, in practice, attaching ourselves to expectations makes little to no sense, because we can't control everything! I suppose you could try, but then you'd just be an overly controlling and neurotic human who plans the fun out of everything and regresses to the emotional state of a toddler when things don't go accordingly. Oh wait...did I just describe someone you know?

This reminds me of a common saying:

LIGHTEN THE FUCK UP OR YOU'RE GOING TO HATE YOURSELF AND EVERYTHING AROUND YOU.

Just kidding.

That is not a common saying, although maybe it should be. The saying actually goes "expectation versus reality equals disappointment."

This saying became a bit of an internet sensation when people started sharing their online purchase fails in the form of memes. You've probably seen them! One part shows what was promised on the website, and the other shows what actually arrived in the mail. For example, the website promises an incredible floor-length gown, dripping in jewels and lace. The delivered product is midcalf length, features two cheap appliqués, and is possibly constructed out of plastic tablecloths. Or my all-time favorite, the beautiful Persian rug. It looked exactly as it had online! It had elaborate details, a deep red color...and was three inches big. Certainly not big enough to cover the floor under a coffee table as per the plans of the person purchasing it...but it *was* to scale with the photo on the website.

The people who made these online purchases were (understandably) very disappointed. They had been promised a very specific thing and had become attached to a clear picture in their head about what they were getting. Then when the package arrived, it was something completely different. The expectations they had were not met, and that picture in their head was shattered, leading to both serious disappointment and hilarious internet fodder.

Some expectations are reasonable. If I order delivery food, I expect it to be hot when it arrives. When my friends make plans to meet me, I expect they will show up (but I know them well enough to expect that half of them will be late). When I order a chai latte, I expect it to be delicious! If these expectations aren't met, I'll certainly be a bit bummed about it, but the consequences aren't terribly serious. I've never heard of anyone being traumatized by a mediocre latte! However, when expectations become unreasonable or attachments become too rigid, the stakes get higher if they're not aligned.

When we place unreasonable expectations on one another, things get messy. An obvious example of this is when parents place too much pressure on their children. That kind of pressure can crack a diamond! Often these kids up rebelling in damaging ways or leading double lives. Toxic relationships of all kinds—familial, friendly, or romantic—are often marked by unreasonable expectations.

When we place rigid expectations on the world outside ourselves, we tend to live life on hold. If you catch yourself frequently thinking in absolutes, you might want to start paying attention to that. Thoughts like "I can be happy when..." or "This is exactly what must happen" can be red flags. The problem with placing expectations outside ourselves is quite simple—we can't control everything! There is a lot that we can do to make our world and the world as a whole as kick-ass as possible. We should want that, and we should advocate for it. But we don't get to dictate every aspect of reality. If your happiness hinges entirely on your expectations being met, you will be routinely disappointed. People who get stuck in this mindset are likely to either become crusty ol' curmudgeons or get trapped in a pit of self-loathing.

The first two forms of expectation (those we place on other people and on the world around us) are easier to spot and compartmentalize because they are outside ourselves; they are separate. The sneakiest and most damaging expectations are often the ones we place on ourselves. Because they are so very *not* separate from us, when we don't meet our own expectations, we end up trapped inside our own heads like prisoners. It fucking sucks. Didn't get the job you interviewed for? Didn't do the thing flawlessly? Made the same mistake again? That's it! Time to flip the table and beat yourself up.

To avoid hurt and disappointment, some people go the route of having decidedly zero expectations in anything or anyone at all. This is different from having a healthy level of nonattachment. Those who say they "just don't give a fuck" often are the ones who give waaaaaaay too many fucks. That apathetic, too-cool-for-school attitude comes from a place of defensive pessimism, and the cost of that defense is high. Instead of risking being hurt and disappointed by the world around them, they guarantee hurting and disappointing themselves. Attachment and expectation, in healthy doses, are necessary. They allow you to map out the plans and goals that give your life personal meaning and direction. Moving forward without them is like bopping around on the ocean in a boat with no sails and no crew. Plus, you're drunk. Also, you mistook your only map for toilet paper.

You've met people who approach life with a defensive, pessimistic, just-don't-give-a-fuck attitude. You've also met people who tackle life in an overcontrolling, too-many-fucks fashion. Although these modes appear to be polar opposites, when you take a closer look, you can see that they are both often rooted in perfectionism. In one, we're desperately clinging to an ideal picture of who we are and what our reality should look like. In the other, we're so afraid of not being able to have our expectations fulfilled that we deny having any attachment to them in the first place. In other words, if it can't be perfect, why bother?

Perfectionism doesn't necessarily have to be a bad word. It can have many positive qualities! Anyone who really hones their craft is a perfectionist. It allows people to dive into the details, really analyzing and breaking them down, and then crank it to eleven. It can separate the okay from the good and the good from the truly excellent. But if it goes too far by setting unrealistically high and unforgiving expectations, perfectionism can quickly become self-sabotage.

For example: perfectionism is a leading cause of people getting caught up in negative cycles of things like dieting or quitting smoking. When people set out to tackle these goals, they have a very clear picture in their head about what they are trying to achieve, and they set strict expectations for themselves. This is all fine and dandy until something goes wrong. Perhaps they fumble the plan or give in to a craving at a party. Then suddenly, they've gone off the deep end because "I already fucked it up!" Time and time again, this leads to yo-yo diets and smoking relapses.

At this point, I gotta come clean with you.

My name is Lindsay Istace, and I am a recovering perfectionist.

When I was a kid, I used to go to summer camp. I loved it! For one whole week, I'd get to be in the woods with my friends. We got to choose different activities for our daily schedules, and I'd always sign up for the same three things: canoeing, archery, and crafts. I was a super creative and art-focused kid, so craft time was serious business to me. I didn't fuck around.

We'd get a new craft project to do every day. While other kids would be chatting and halfheartedly stringing together friendship bracelets, I'd still be at the supplies table stressing about the perfect color combination. At the end of the hour, the other kids would leave with a handful of bracelets while my singular bracelet would be left in the craft room unfinished. I'd always tell myself that I would finish it tomorrow, but the next day, there would be a new project to work on.

You see where this is going. By the end of the week, my friends would have a bunch of things that they had completed and could be proud of. Meanwhile, I (cue the sad violin music) would have a shoe-box of half-finished projects that caused me unreasonable amounts of shame and anxiety.

The last year I attended camp, things got even worse. On the first day of crafts, we were given a painting project. The project was simple and only had two steps: Select rock. Paint rock. Done! Sounds easy, right? Well, for me, it wasn't. Before I picked a rock, I had to decide exactly what I wanted to paint. It was going to be a beautiful land-scape, inspired by the humbly scenic drive I experienced every year from the back seat of my grandfather's truck on the way to camp. In my mind, I can still see the image I wanted to paint. It's beautiful. It gives me a warm feeling of comfort, reminding me of the sense of care-free adventure and awe that is experienced so effortlessly in youth.

If I had ever finished painting that damn rock, then maybe I could show you! Instead, I spent half of the first day deciding what to paint and the other half picking out the right rock and paint colors. The rest of the week I spent painting while the other kids completed new proj-ects daily. I fretted over every stroke of the paintbrush and stressed about whether the trees had enough realistic depth and texture. By the end of the week, my rock was the only project I took home. It was about 40 percent of the way to the grand vision I had in mind. I took that rock home and swore I would finish it. But for whatever reason *cough* crippling perfectionism *cough cough* it was never completed.

My perfectionism used to be a serious problem. Every project I started was doomed from the beginning, no matter what it was. It could be creating practical organizational systems, developing healthy habits, making art, or learning a new skill. I had my expectations set so high that nothing stood a chance. I would overanalyze everything, trying to make it absolutely and undeniably perfect, as though perfection was a universally objective and tangible state. I'd waste so much of my time and energy that I'd run out of time and energy before I could produce anything that looked vaguely complete. Then I'd be forced to put it aside unfinished, joining the ever-growing pile of incomplete projects that haunted me. Every. Fucking. Time.

Over the years, I have put some serious mental energy into my relationship with perfectionism. I've become much better at letting go and setting reasonable expectations. I've stopped clinging so desperately to goals and allowed myself to become more flexible in them. Now, (most of the time) when I start slipping back into old cycles, I can catch myself and pause. Inhale the Good Shit. Exhale the Bullshit. And move on. As a result, I actually accomplish more of what I set out to do, and I'm less afraid to do things in the first place. The biggest perk, although it seems so simple that it might sound silly, is that I'm finally just nicer to myself!

Things like perfectionism, crippling expectations, and rigid ideals all come from the same place: fear. This wild world we live in is full of uncertainty. Nothing ever remains permanently still or balanced; it's all in a constant state of change. In both our internal and external worlds, nothing is ever decidedly finished or perfect. Add a dash of existential dread on top of all that and BOOM! It can be scary as hell. It's 110 percent understandable why fear then makes us want to cling to absolute ideals and expectations: they promise shelter. Unfortunately, those promises are just Bullshit empty mirages. If we can—even if only for moments at a time—find the courage to lean in to the chaos and anarchy, we can find the beauty in it. Rather than getting overwhelmed and swept away in temporary details, letting go of inflexible ideals and expectations allows us to find some of that "contentment in the present."

The trick to handling expectations isn't to stop having them. The trick is to develop a healthy relationship with them. We already know that giving decidedly zero fucks is unhealthy. On the other end of the scale, giving every conceivable fuck about everything we could conceivably give a fuck about is debilitating...and is also unhealthy. There is a lot of space in the middle of that scale where we can find balance. The health of our fucks is important! One easy way to care for them is to manage how we react when things don't go well. This is an important skill to develop because, let's be real, at some point, we will find outcomes falling short of our expectations and face disappointment and failure. It's part of life! But the big question is, what do you do when this happens?

A.   Freeze like a startled baby deer.
B.   Flip. The fuck. Out!
C.   Pretend that you never cared in the first place.

D.   Store the memory deep down so your mind can pull it out sporadically to remind you that you (and everything around you) are terrible.

E.   All of the above.

F.   None of the above.

I'm going to go out on a limb and say that we've all at some point reacted with at least one of the first five options. Me too. No judgment here. But what if, instead of self-sabotaging or throwing a fit, we moved on in a constructive way?

You can hold yourself accountable for failure and unmet expectations without crucifying yourself. You can face disappointment and hurt caused by the actions of others or the less-than-ideal outcomes of events. You can also lean in to the chaos to take positive aspects away from these things, which will make you stronger for the future. Doing so will help you on your life's journey. And you'll find it to be a helpful guideline in your journey to becoming Zen as fuck.

BREATHE IN THE GOOD SHIT.

Take in the lessons learned and the experience points gained.

    Give yourself credit for your courage and strength.

BREATHE OUT THE BULLSHIT.

Make room for something better.

Be willing to let go of less-than-awesome pains, patterns, fears, and habits.

Breathe. Give yourself some love, you majestic badass!
Get up and get ready to move on.

One more time, badass! Inhale the Good Shit. Exhale the Bullshit. Your breath will be a superpower on your Rage Yoga journey. Let it bring in the things you want and let go of the things you don't want to hold on to. Let it reinforce both your mind and body.

So whaddya say? Should we put this into action?
Fuck yeah.

🔥 BREATH AND MOVEMENT SEQUENCE

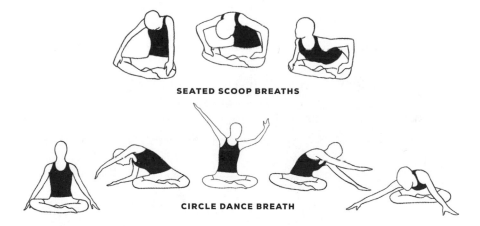

SEATED SCOOP BREATHS

CIRCLE DANCE BREATH

Sit your ass down and get comfy. Hang out here for a couple breaths, feeling the air come and go. Feel your lungs expand and your shoulders rise on the inhale. Feel your chest and shoulders fall on the exhale. Next, begin Scoop Breaths. Put your hands onto your knees and "scoop" your body forward, following your inhale. Finish your inhale as your chest rises. Lower your head as you curl your back, letting your next exhale push you backward. Repeat this five times, scooping on your inhale and curling on your exhale, then return to your neutral sitting position. Prepare for Circle Dance Breath! On your next inhale, letting your breath do as much of the lifting as possible, bring one arm up and over to the other side of your body. Let your exhale move your body, using the engagement of your abdominal muscles, as your arms sweep from this side of your body to the other. Repeat five times each way.

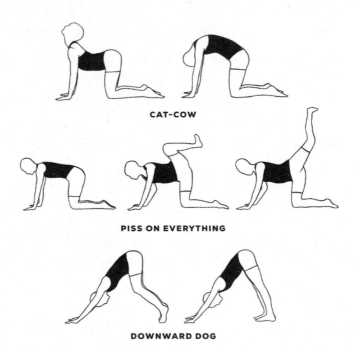

CAT-COW

PISS ON EVERYTHING

DOWNWARD DOG

Come into a neutral position on all fours. It's Cat-Cow time! Inhale to Cow, letting your chest fill with air as it lifts up and your gaze moves to the ceiling. Exhale to Cat, using the force of your exhale to arch your back. Repeat five times, allowing your breath to take the lead. When you're done, Piss on Everything! Lift one leg, then...get curious! As your breath comes and goes, how does it connect with your leg? Play around with this leg for seven breaths, then repeat on the other side. When you're done, return to your neutral position on all fours and curl your toes under so they point to the front of your mat. Pause. Breathe in the Good Shit. Let it soak in. Exhale the Bullshit. Use the force of this breath to engage your core, ground down through your arms and legs, and rise (like the majestic badass you are) into Downward Dog. Stay here for five breaths.

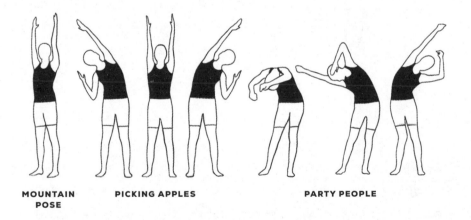

MOUNTAIN POSE   **PICKING APPLES**   **PARTY PEOPLE**

Follow that badass breath as you step, or hop or dance, into Mountain Pose. Stay here for three breaths while paying attention to how they move and feel throughout your body. When you're ready, commence Picking Apples. Let your inhale lengthen your arms overhead, making them feel light. Use the exhale to keep your core muscles strong while you bend to one side, reaching up and over. As it fills your chest, allow your inhale to bring your body back to center before exhaling to the other side. Repeat five times and prepare for Party People! Trust your breath as it encourages you to sway, bend, and move all around. Party for seven breaths.

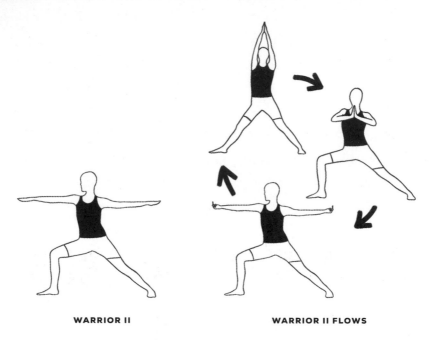

WARRIOR II   **WARRIOR II FLOWS**

As you let your next inhale lift you, shift your weight into one foot. Use the strength of your exhale to step the lifted foot back into Warrior II. Feel fierce as fuck in this pose for three breaths. Next, move into Warrior II Flows. On your inhale, straighten your front leg and let your arms rise overhead, giving yourself a well-deserved high five. On your exhale, bring your hands down to your chest and bend the front leg as you powerfully return to Warrior II. Repeat three times.

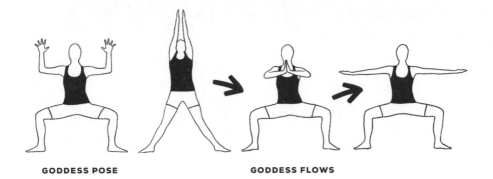

GODDESS POSE　　　　　　　　　　**GODDESS FLOWS**

As you exhale, use the extra engagement of your muscles to stay balanced as you turn your body open to the side of your mat. Revel in this grounding force as you breathe in, then, as you breathe out, bend your knees as you sink into Goddess Pose for three breaths. Moving into Goddess Flows, use your inhale to lift and lengthen as you straighten your knees and give yourself a high five overhead. Exhale as you descend, strong and in control, while bending your knees and bringing your arms back down, then out to return to Goddess Pose. Repeat three times.

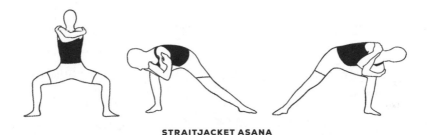

STRAITJACKET ASANA

Give yourself a hug! You deserve it. Reach your arms across your body to grab the opposite side shoulders. Inhale here. On your exhale, slowly curve and lower your upper body and come into Straitjacket Asana.

Follow as the breath leads your body.

Just. Follow.

Allow it to sway you...

Lifting and lowering...

Bending and twisting...

There is no right or wrong.

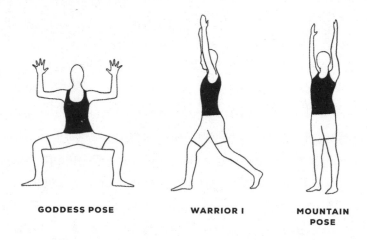

GODDESS POSE   **WARRIOR I**   **MOUNTAIN POSE**

Let your inhale lift you back up as you return to Goddess Pose. Take a breath to ground your Badass Self here. Use the power of your next exhale to steady yourself as you (ever so slightly) lift your heels and shift your weight onto the balls of your feet. Rotate your body toward the front of your mat as you come into Warrior I. Take three breaths here, you wonderful warrior. Let your knees bend slightly on your next inhale. On the following exhale, shift your weight to balance on your front foot as you bring the back leg forward, stepping into Mountain Pose. Inhale those hands up overhead. Exhale them down to the center of your chest and give yourself a solid "fuck yeah!"

Forgiveness and Letting Go

No matter how much of a badass we are, at the end of the day, we are still just humans. Not just you and me, no! Everyone on this whimsically wonderful (and sometimes terrifying) planet. No amount of ass kicking or stardust or unicorn farts is going to change how very human we are. This has some upsides. For one, I am a big fan of opposable thumbs. We are also some of the only animals who have an acute sense of musicality and who have sex as a leisure activity. So that's neat! But being human also means that we are inevitably going to fuck up. In this lifetime, it's going to happen more than once. In fact, it's going to happen a lot. Beyond simply fucking up, human beings hurt one another. Sometimes the hurt is small, like an innocent misunderstanding. But sometimes that hurt is caused by a serious, potentially compounding transgression that leaves us wondering...how can someone be such a dick?

Between our genetics and the circumstances we're raised in, everyone has a story that influences the way they think and act. It can be really hard to understand why people do the shit they do, but everyone is really just doing the best they can to survive and thrive. The methods that people use to do so are often informed by their own traumas and Bullshit, and those methods can cause harm. We can have a role in deciding to what degree our predetermined factors and histories control us. Some people do the continuous work that it takes, even though it's never completely finished or perfect, which allows them to break cycles of hurt. Some never learn that it's possible, because they are stuck just trying to survive. And then there are some who, quite frankly, are just assholes. Look, just because yoga is all about love and unity, doesn't mean I'm going to candy-coat humanity and sing "Kumbaya." Some people are legitimately malicious. Good people can still cause hurt, but usually it comes from a place of ignorance, not malice. Either way, the old cliché is true: hurt people hurt people.

The ability to forgive is a trait of a badass. When we don't forgive, we get stuck in cycles of Bullshit because we can't let go of that pain. And again, hurt people hurt people, so then we become partly responsible for perpetuating the cycle. This isn't meant to come across as victim blaming; it's simply a fact that holding on to pain creates real trauma. This then becomes part of our personal baggage, which gains a level of control over us by informing our thoughts and actions. Forgiveness is key to freeing us from this cycle so that we can move forward without lugging around extra Bullshit.

Forgiveness is the act of extending enough empathy and compassion to someone to understand that they are human and they're just doing their best to survive and thrive, even if their best can be shitty. It's a baller move! Yet we often have backward beliefs about what its real purpose is. Forgiveness is not designed for the person who caused the harm to be able to move past it. That's done through reparation and making amends, both of which are vast and important topics of their own. Forgiveness is really for the person giving it. Its purpose is to help you move past it so you can avoid getting caught up in Bullshit cycles. Forgiving someone doesn't mean you've waved a magic wand and suddenly everything is fucking sunshine and rainbows. People are still accountable for their actions, and when someone hurts you, the wounds are still real and valid! Forgiveness is what helps keep them from getting infected. Even though sometimes scars remain, most wounds can heal completely over time.

Still, some things are much easier to forgive than others. It can be easy when the transgression isn't astronomical or when it has clearly taken place out of ignorance and not malice. But it can be really fucking hard, maybe even impossible, to muster compassion and empathy to forgive someone who has deeply hurt you or those you care about. And honestly, we all probably have much better things to do than strain a muscle trying to empathize with assholes! A basic understanding that they're just people who are hurt in their own ways and who are trapped in their own Bullshit cycles can be enough.

Since forgiveness is designed for the person giving it, you get to choose what it looks like. For small stuff, this can be pretty easy. Big stuff can be much harder. One-size-fits-all clothing is un-fucking-realistic 99 percent of the time, and forgiveness is not a one-size-fits-all thing. You can forgive while maintaining your boundaries or establishing new ones. Rebuilding trust with someone who has violated yours isn't mandatory at all either. Those heavy conversations can sometimes be impossible or cause more pain than they can heal. Again, *you get to choose what forgiveness looks like for you.* It's something that you do for yourself, not for those who caused you pain. Sometimes that means that forgiveness is healthiest when it happens internally, without the need to reach out and engage with dickheads. It's all about you not having to carry around extra baggage or get caught up in someone else's Bullshit cycles.

 ## KAPALABHATI BREATH

The thoughts and emotions that pass through our heads and hearts can be difficult to sort out. Sometimes they get knotted and sticky! You can use something like a *kapalabhati* breath practice to shake it up and get these stubborn fuckers unstuck.

Traditionally, this breath is used to cleanse yourself of stale air and energy that is stagnating in you. It kicks your lungs into high gear and gives you some extra invigorating energy. It's helpful when you're feeling bogged down and need a mental reset.

Step 1: Blow your nose! Otherwise, you may be picking boogers up off your mat.

Step 2: Find a comfortable seated position and settle in. Take a couple of natural deep breaths. Close your eyes. When you're ready, let your next exhale out quickly through your nose in a series of sharp bursts. Use your abdominal muscles to stutter these bursts and push the air out. Take your time with your inhale, relaxing your abdominal muscles and letting it come in passively through your nose. Make your inhale much longer than your exhale.

Do this eleven times for three rounds. Take your time between these rounds, observing how your body and mind feel after each round. If you find yourself feeling light-headed, take some natural breaths and as much time as you need before continuing on with the next round.

Once things have been shaken up, let's see if we can get moving them again! This is a great time to let out some of the backed-up crap. It's tempting to make the obvious poop joke here, but I'm going to save that for the time being... In the meantime, let's let some shit go!

LET THAT SHIT GO BREATH

Get yourself in a standing position, starting off in a strong Mountain Pose.

Now it's time to let that shit go! Stay grounded in your legs as you allow your upper body to fall, aggressively flopping down. Surrender to the whims of gravity, letting your arms swing in a rag-doll-like fashion. Exhale through your mouth, and get vocal about it! You might let out an incoherent grumble or maybe even a full sentence of pent-up Bullshit that you just need to get off your chest.

Once you've successfully let that shit go, stay in that folded position, letting your upper body and neck hang heavy. Find some stillness here, or play around with whatever movement feels good. When you're ready, take a slight bend in your knees, and begin stacking your weight over your center of gravity. Rolling up one vertebra at a time, use the force of your breath to build yourself up tall again. As your chest rolls up, take a nice big inhale of all that Good Shit, and bring your arms overhead. On your exhale, repeat this loud and aggressive flopping. Let it out! Let. That. Shit. Go.

Repeat three to five times.

Although forgiveness is designed for the person extending it, the hardest person to forgive can often be ourselves. We don't always do the right thing, and sometimes, even if we do "the right thing," causing pain to ourselves or others is unavoidable. We've all done things that we are not proud of, and they can be hard to let go. It can make you feel trapped inside your own head, unable to escape the person who's pissing you off. It can be tempting to numb yourself to it, because even if it's a cycle of self-sabotage, picking up a bottle can be easier than facing your own shit. If we don't process these feelings in a healthy way, though, they can fester and mutate until they're barely recognizable. They can eat away at our mental and emotional health, becoming sticky emotional knots of guilt, shame, anger, and anxiety.

To some extent, we all have that nagging voice in the backs of our heads. You know the one. It pulls us out of the present to remind us why we should believe that we are just the fucking worst and everything is shit. Call it what you want: your inner critic, monkey thoughts, self-doubt, whatever. I call mine Agatha.

Agatha is the anxious voice in my head, popping up to remind me that I'm a piece of human garbage. She'll remind me of anything I've done wrong just in case I forgot. Sometimes it's serious, like causing legitimate hurt to someone I loved. Sometimes it's not, like that one thing I said to someone at a party six years ago that may have been perceived as condescending, although I meant it as a compliment. In the past, Agatha has even taken positive memories and twisted them into stories about why I should hate myself and everything is hopeless.

When I noticed this pattern in myself, I tried to catch those thoughts and change them. But it happened so often that I got really frustrated, and then I'd say things to myself like "dammit, Lindsay! Why are you such a bitch to yourself?!" I didn't like the fact that by scolding myself for having these anxious thoughts in the first place, I was claiming full responsibility for them. But I wasn't actively choosing them. They were the result of Bullshit that I had collected for years that was now subconsciously bubbling up to the surface in the form of anxiety. They were not the result of me consciously digging into my personal cellar of memories to find something to beat myself with. Plus, being a bitch to myself for being a bitch to myself wasn't helpful; it was just a negative feedback loop. To break that loop, I decided to make the voice separate from me. So I named it.

When Agatha is being a real big jerk, I'll even say "Hey, Nag-atha! It's going to be okay. I know that you're just trying to look out for me in some sick way, but you're not helping." Or "Yo, Agatha, if you can't be nice, you're not invited today!" Nine times out of ten, Agatha quiets right down.

FRIENDLY REMINDER: YOU ARE ENOUGH. YOU ARE WORTHY OF SELF-LOVE AND FORGIVENESS.

Cut yourself some slack already! You will do better, even if just incrementally, in the future. Keep learning from your mistakes, and give yourself credit when you improve. If you've done something wrong, you can be accountable for your actions without crucifying yourself. Sometimes you can carry feelings of guilt or shame that have been put on you by the actions of others. No matter how you have accumulated Bullshit, you deserve to heal from that, and it begins with giving yourself patience, understanding, and forgiveness.

> **JUST BREATHE. IF YOU CAN BREATHE, YOU CAN GET THROUGH DAMN NEAR ANYTHING.**

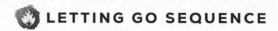

LETTING GO SEQUENCE

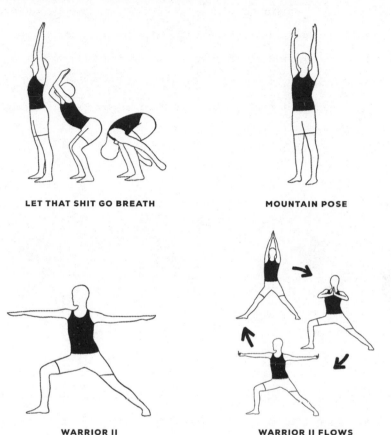

LET THAT SHIT GO BREATH

MOUNTAIN POSE

WARRIOR II

WARRIOR II FLOWS

Stand at the top of your mat and check in with yourself. What is it that you want to let go of? It can be something specific or it can be something that you can't quite put into words. It can be one thing or many things. Whatever the hell it is, when you're ready, inhale the Good Shit as you take your hands overhead and begin Let That Shit Go Breath. Let. It. Go! Repeat three times and then come into Mountain Pose. Having just expelled a bunch of Bullshit, stay here for three breaths, bringing in new Good Shit on every inhale. Exhale, stepping back into Warrior II and gazing confidently over your front middle finger. If it feels good, turn that middle finger up! Stay strong here for three breaths. Next, begin Warrior II Flows. Complete this flow five times. Notice the easy strength that comes with your inhales. As your arms straighten back out to Warrior II, use your exhales to release any stale Bullshit that's holding on.

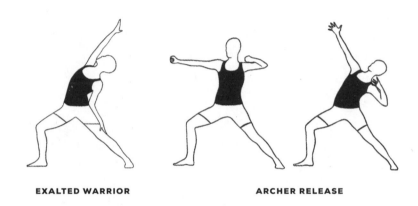

EXALTED WARRIOR   **ARCHER RELEASE**

Exhale, engaging your core as you lean back. Then inhale, lifting your front arm up and over, coming into Exalted Warrior. Hold this pose, heroic as fuck, for three breaths. Moving into Archer Release, inhale as you string your imaginary bow with whatever Bullshit you so choose. Then let it go! Let your exhale be sharp and loud as you shoot your bow to send it far away. Repeat three times, noticing any sensations that may pop up with each release. You might feel warmer, stronger, or lighter.

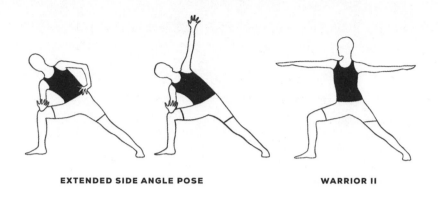

EXTENDED SIDE ANGLE POSE　　　**WARRIOR II**

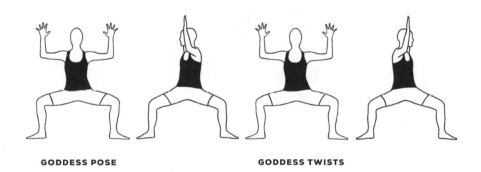

GODDESS POSE　　　**GODDESS TWISTS**

Bring your front arm forward, resting your elbow on your front knee, as you come into Side Angle Pose. Hold this for three breaths, grounding through your legs and lifting with your core. Inhale the Good Shit, letting it reinforce you. Exhale the Bullshit, letting go of what you longer need. Inhale to Warrior II. You know what to do—gaze confidently over your front middle finger and, if it feels good, turn that middle finger up! Hold this for three breaths. Rise up onto the balls of your feet and lift your heels as you exhale, turning slowly to the open side of your mat and coming into Goddess Pose. Like the unshakable badass that you are, stay here for three breaths. Commence Goddess Twists! Take a strong breath in, then let it out, sharp and loud, as you twist to one side. Let your body unwind naturally as you inhale slowly. Once back to center, repeat this sharp exhale and twist to the other side. Repeat, twisting each way five times.

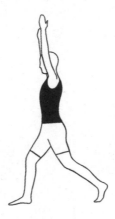

WARRIOR I

Rise onto the balls of your feet as you turn toward the front of your mat, exhaling into Warrior I. Pause here, noticing any sensations, thoughts, or feelings that might pop up. They could be comfortable things, such as feeling grounded, strong, or relieved. They could also be uncomfortable things, like feeling anxious, weak, or sad. If this is the case, then don't try to change these feelings or get judgy with them. Letting go is a process. Feeling is a part of that process...even when it sucks! A warrior isn't a person without fear. A warrior is a person who is brave despite their fear. Whatever it is that you're feeling here, you can be strong in it. Breathe in the Good Shit, exhale the Bullshit. Stay here for three to five breaths.

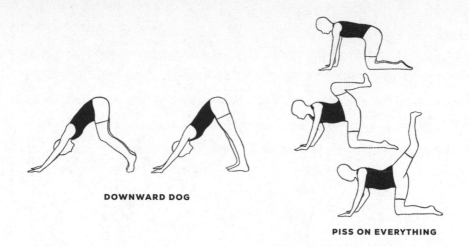

DOWNWARD DOG

PISS ON EVERYTHING

Exhale, lengthening your spine and engaging your core, as you bend your knees and bring your hands to the mat on either side of your front foot. Step this foot back and come into Downward Dog. Stay here for three breaths. Next, lower down onto your knees and Piss on Everything. Kick your leg out, or swing it in circles, or imagine urinating on a steaming pile of Bullshit that has been weighing you down. Whatever you do, do what feels good, and let it go! Continue to Piss on Everything for three to five breaths.

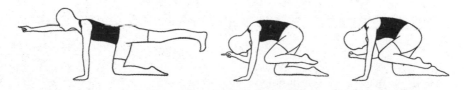

MOTHER FUCKIN' UNICORN

Oh hell yeah! It's time to be a majestic Mother Fuckin' Unicorn. Inhale as you curve your back, bringing one knee and your opposite side elbow together underneath you. Exhale, sending the lifted arm and leg out long. Repeat. Inhale, bringing in all of that Good Shit (including your lifted arm and leg) and holding it tight under you. Let it soak into you. You might even imagine it breaking apart the Bullshit that is hard to let go of, loosening its grip and softening its edges. Exhale that Bullshit. Let it the fuck go as you extend your arm and leg, once again resuming your natural form as a badass beast. Be a Mother Fuckin' Unicorn for five breaths.

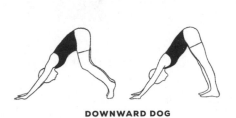

DOWNWARD DOG

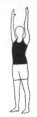

MOUNTAIN POSE

Inhale, curling your toes under you and toward the top of your mat. Exhale, engaging your core and straightening your arms to come into Downward Dog. Hold this pose for three breaths. Inhale, taking a slight bend at the knees and elbows. Exhale, using the extra core engagement to either step or hop both feet up to your hands. Next, slowly roll your body up into Mountain Pose. Inhale and lift your hands up high overhead, then exhale as you bring them down to the center of your chest. Give yourself a solid "fuck yeah!"

So, badass, I wanna ask you some questions. Take your time. There's no rush. You don't need to have all the answers right now. Ready? Here we go.

- What are your breathing habits like? Do you often find yourself holding it or taking shallow breaths?
- Are you open and ready for the Good Shit?

- **✗** Do you hold on to Bullshit? Is there anything in particular that is hard to let go of?

- **✗** How do you deal when shit doesn't go your way? Are the fucks you give healthy?

- **✗** Do you feel that others have unreasonable or inflexible expectations of you? Do you have any for other people and the world around you? How about for yourself?

- **✗** Do you find yourself living in the past or future so often that you forget the present?

- **✗** Is there forgiveness you're withholding, for someone else or for yourself?

- **✗** Do you have an inner critic or anxious voice that is too loud too often?

Nobody wants to climb up Mount Everest with shoes full of pebbles or a backpack full of bricks! Do your best to take that shit out, learn what you can from it, and then leave it at base camp. As you begin this Rage Yoga journey, be willing and ready to let go. Free up as much space as possible in your metaphorical backpack to make room for something new. Let's do this!

IT BEGINS WITH A BREATH. INHALE THE GOOD SHIT. EXHALE THE BULLSHIT.

Can I get a "Fuck yeah!"?

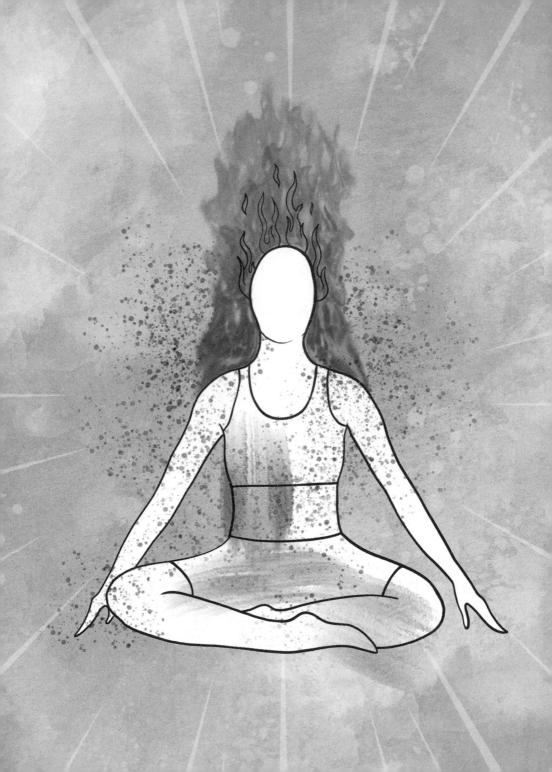

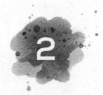

THE POWER OF
STILLNESS

> **"If you're having a stressed-out day, remember the sloth. They don't do shit, and they haven't gone extinct. I'm sure you can afford to take a nap."**
> **—ZE FRANK IN *TRUE FACTS ABOUT SLOTHS***

We live in a fast-paced world that celebrates success and accomplishment. At a glance, that makes a lot of sense, right? What're we going to praise otherwise? Typos and apathy?

WTF Is Success?

We celebrate people who win and make big things happen. We reward those who excel and innovate. So everyone wants to be successful! Now we have millions of people running around on the quest for success, flailing like those wacky, waving, inflatable-arm tube men you see at car dealerships. They're setting goals, going to meetings, making appointments, laying down plans, and staying super busy in general. But why?

We've been told that success is constantly moving forward and achieving. Between the lines of that narrative is a dangerous one: being successful means being busy!

The idea that being busy equates to success is easy to buy into. If you're busy, then you're obviously getting stuff done! The busier you are, the more ass you must be kicking. Your time is in demand. *You fucking matter.* But that mode of thinking can lead you into a trap.

When we fall into the busy trap, our bodies flood with tension. We start treating them as though they are hollow husks to be abused in order to reach our destinations. It leads to us switching to autopilot and clinging to our busy schedules for some sense of control and meaning. Life ends up living us instead of the other way around. Our minds start running away from us like caffeinated toddlers in a department store. We get so goddamn overloaded that we can't hear ourselves think. Those caffeinated asshole toddlers begin screaming.

So many people have fallen into the busy trap that we've collectively fucked ourselves and silently rewritten the definition for the word *success*.

SUCCESS (NOUN)

1. being very busy being important and making as much money as possible

Because of this, people everywhere are in the busy trap, grinding through bloated to-do lists of tedious Bullshit in an attempt to claim some small corner of success. They're overwhelming themselves in an attempt to find a sense of importance and distract themselves from a growing feeling of disconnect. Look, I'm not saying that everyone who claims to be busy is full of shit. I'm saying that the definition of success that we have come to know as true, even if only subconsciously, is toxic.

Now let's take a second to look at what *Merriam-Webster's Dictionary* has to say about the definition of success.

SUCCESS (NOUN)

1. degree or measure of succeeding
2. favorable or desired outcome
3. one that succeeds

Sounds way more healthy, right? This definition is one that leaves room for us to play and decide what we really want instead of what we've been told we should want. None of this is to say that you should burn your to-do list or decide to give up on your lofty ambitions. But there is a way that you can succeed more by doing less...and release a ton of the Bullshit that you've started to store up in your brain and body while you're at it!

To get the ball rolling, I asked a bunch of people how they personally defined success. Here's a sample of some of the responses I got back:

* "Being where you want to be, or at least on the path toward it."

- ✕ "Finishing an entire plate of poutine without spilling gravy on my pants!"
- ✕ "Following your passions while being there for those who need you."
- ✕ "Money."
- ✕ "Waking up without the feeling of stress or anxiety."
- ✕ "If you can honestly say you are happy in life, then you have succeeded."
- ✕ "Being able to buy coffee!"
- ✕ "Making goals and doing what you can to achieve them. If you don't reach them, it's okay. Success is trying over and over again until you feel satisfied with your outcome."
- ✕ "Success is clearly defining your goals, achieving them, and still being able to live with yourself once you are there."
- ✕ "An unlimited amount of bacon."

As you can see, these answers are all very different. Some are silly and some are more serious. Either way, there are three common threads, and each answer has at least one of them:

1. A sense of purpose and the ability to affect change.
2. Freedom from worry about things such as money and time.
3. Finding contentment in the present.

Now it's your turn. What does success mean to you? You don't have to answer this right away. When you ask yourself a question like this, your subconscious may take its sweet-ass time, but it will always give you the answer. You just need to wait and listen. If nothing is jumping out at you, don't worry about it. You're not broken. This is tricky shit! You can start by making some simple notes below. Come back to it later if you need to.

TO ME, SUCCESS MEANS:

When we define success for ourselves, it becomes easier to chill the fuck out and prioritize our lives in a more meaningful way. The more we take this personal definition to heart, the easier it becomes to let go of junk we cling to that isn't actually important. When we let that shit go, we suddenly have extra fucks to give to the things that really matter! It's amazing how much happier and genuinely productive we are when we're not just busy!

When you break it down, life is really just a wild RPG (role-playing game) that has gotten out of control. This new definition of success is essentially a guideline for how you play. It's like you've gone into the settings menu and changed some of the parameters of the game. When you do that, it cuts down the excess of mind-numbing side quests that make it feel more like an obligation than a game, and it gives you a clearer map to play with.

Is my nerd showing? Sorry, not sorry.

When we redefine success for ourselves, we bust through the idea that we have to *constantly* be active (mentally/physically/whatever-ly) in order to matter. Suddenly, we have the energy to focus on the things that really light us up. It becomes easier to understand ourselves and to revel in the power of stillness. Soon, we find that we can do more with less perceived work, and in the long run, we are more successful for it.

At this point, you're probably either giddy with excitement or waiting for me to sell you snake oil. If you're in the second camp, I get it. How can rewiring your conceptions of one word and doing fewer things make you a better, more productive, and happier human? Stick with me, you majestic badass. We're just getting to the good stuff.

Meditation

All this can be done with meditation.

Now I know that some people reading this may have just rolled their eyes at me. Meditation can often be thrown under the bus for being really "hippie-dippie." I've also heard many people say that it's absurd to try to achieve an empty mind, because after all, "isn't the point of having a brain to think?"

The truth is that most of our thinking isn't exactly top quality. This is true even for the biggest, juiciest, most thinkiest brains! The average attention span is so short that most people can only truly concentrate on any one thing for a couple of seconds at a time. We're flooded with a buttload of thoughts at any given moment and are barely aware of most of them. Trying to pick them out individually can be like trying to use chopsticks to pick up a single grain of rice from a bowl while blindfolded. It's chaotic, it's messy, and we can all agree that it's inefficient as fuck. So instead of stubbornly forcing our brains to work as hard as they can *all the fucking time*, why not take a rest?

Meditation is so much more than just a rest. If you go to the gym and pump iron like a boss, you see changes in your body. Your muscles get stronger, and you may even discover new ones you never knew you had! Meditating is like pumping iron for your brain. With enough time and practice, you can develop impressive, rippling brain muscles. They're not the kind of muscles you can flex at the beach, but they sure as hell come with sweet benefits.

By draining the messy bogs that choke our minds, meditation allows us to use our heads in a way that is *actually* productive. It improves memory and the ability to concentrate and can go a long way in assisting with mental health. It keeps our Bullshit baggage lighter by making it easier to process intense emotions or events. With the extra mental control and bandwidth that we gain, challenging problems, projects, and life dramas become easier to tackle. Basically, we start to fire on all cylinders, more often and for longer periods of time, allowing us to *kick all the ass for real.*

As an extra badass bonus, meditation also does wonders for the body! It is a wildly effective tool for reducing and managing stress. It's probably for this reason that it's often credited with assisting in things like regulating sleep patterns and lowering blood pressure. Many studies have even found meditation helpful in pain management, which makes sense, since our bodies perceive pain more acutely when in a state of stress. It's not a magic cure-all, but it is a natural, free, and highly effective tool that you can use anywhere at any time. And that sounds pretty fucking magical to me!

When most people picture mediation, they picture an intensely religious affair. Maybe there are some candles and incense or stoic, robed figures hanging around. Maybe some light panpipes or Gregorian chanting. Sure, that can be mediation. But it doesn't have to be *your* mediation, unless you're into that sort of thing! There are many different kinds of mediation, just like there are many different kinds of people. Chances are that one of them will fit you.

The first kind of meditation that I want to talk about, the kind that I'll mostly be focusing on in this chapter, is all about thought observation. When I was first introduced to thought observation as a form of meditation, I found it tough to grasp. Wrapping my head around it was like trying to get a grip on a greased-up pig. It sounded both difficult and like an absurd waste of time. Then it was described to me in a much more graphic way, and suddenly it clicked (although I was a little grossed out). So I hope you're not eating, because we're going to get a little nasty.

Take a Shit with Your Brain

Pooping is good for you! If you don't take a dump for several days, then you don't feel so hot. You might not even realize why right away, but you'll start to get a little twitchy. You become more introverted, lethargic, and irrational because you're in genuine discomfort. It's hard to get anything done, and you don't feel like yourself at all. Instead, you slowly become a grumpy shit demon.

A mind left to its own devices will run around aimlessly. Our thoughts become like those unsupervised, caffeinated toddlers that we talked about earlier, running in wild circles, into walls, and into one another. They're like hell spawn. You can't tell them apart from one another, and for some reason, they keep multiplying! When the mind becomes this chaotic, it gets bogged down. Just like you and I do with overloaded bowels, the mind becomes a grumpy shit demon.

JUST LIKE OUR BOWELS NEED TO EMPTY, WE NEED TO TAKE A SHIT... WITH OUR BRAINS!

Most of the thoughts we have throughout the day *are* shit! Harsh to hear? Well, it's true. Again, sorry, not sorry. Most of the thoughts we have throughout the day are thanks to our "monkey brains." This part of the brain is responsible for the mindless chatter that constantly happens upstairs, whether we hear it or not. It's constantly reminding, observing, and remarking on everything in our past, present, and future. It. Talks. Constantly. The monkey brain doesn't have many intelligent thoughts. These are the thoughts that our survival instincts give us, because on some genetic level, our brains still think we live in the jungle and that danger is around every corner. The thoughts and fears that our monkey brains yammer on about are their attempts to protect us from danger. When we first started walking on two legs, these thoughts were important. They kept us alert and safe. In modern times, we generally don't need them, but they don't know that. They're just trying to help, desperately serving their function when they're no longer functional. In fact, the poor things don't realize that all their hard work just makes our day-to-day lives more difficult.

A lot of us have a hard time letting go of these thoughts and moving past the monkey brain, which is understandable. It can be hard and downright scary! Because of how loud it is, the monkey brain often keeps us distracted from the real workings of our minds. When we're distracted, we don't feel the weight of the bogs choking our minds. We don't see the stuff trapped in them.

It can also be hard to let go of these monkey brain thoughts because we often find a sense of identity in them. A yoga teacher of mine once compared this to a light bulb saying, "I am electricity." That would be freakin' ridiculous. First of all, holy shit, a talking light bulb! Second, a light bulb is not made of the electric current that runs through it. In a similar way, monkey brain thoughts run through us. We have more control over the whole situation than a light bulb does, but we do have one thing in common: while they may be the most immediately impactful parts of us, we are made up of more than just what passes through us.

Back to taking a shit with your brain!

Holding on to these monkey brain thoughts is a lot like holding in your poop.

Don't hold in your poop. That's gross and bad for you!

Releasing your bowels regularly is important to stay in good health. The same thing is true about releasing your monkey brain thoughts. Holding them in is going to lead to some serious mental constipation. It's time to *let that shit go!* This mental bowel movement can be urged along with the use of thought observation in meditation.

Meditation happens in the space between daydreaming and concentrating. When you daydream, you let your mind float along carelessly from one thing to another. When you concentrate, you hold your attention on one thing and do not allow it to wander. So when you practice thought observation as a form of meditation, you let your mind wander in one spot. This spot is your metaphorical mind crapper, and it's where you can unload those backed-up brain bowels. Your job is to simply sit and let any thoughts or feelings that arise be like turds. Allow them to pass through you, plop out of you, and then be over. In this space between daydreaming and concentrating, you don't fixate on turds or let your mind get carried away by them. You wouldn't drop a literal shit and then pick it up out of the toilet, would you? You just experience it as it passes and let it go.

If you haven't taken a mind shit in a while, or ever, then you'll be backed up. You'll find that there are a lot of thought dumps, some very difficult to pass, or perhaps even a constant stream. This is really common when you first begin the practice of thought observation. It makes sense, right? You've probably got a lot of that monkey brain Bullshit stored up in there. But if you keep sitting down and doing the work to empty the backlog, you'll notice a shift. The thought dumps become easier to pass, and the empty spaces between those turds become longer. In that emptiness, you'll find some powerful stillness, and this stillness is why we come to the mind crapper.

If poop grosses you out, you're missing out on an analogy that I think is both hilarious and on point, but I respect your preferences. Instead, you can try thinking about your mind like an empty screen. Any thoughts that you have show up on the screen like movie credits. But that's all they are. They pop up, you notice them, and they move on without you following them.

THOUGHT OBSERVATION MEDITATION

Find a comfortable position to sit or lie down.

Set a timer. If you're new to meditation, try a shorter session of three to five minutes. If you're feeling adventurous, try ten minutes.

As you begin, close and relax your eyes.

Let your breathing come naturally without trying to control or change it.

Take a moment to ease into stillness. Just chill. The. Fuck. Out.

Bring your attention to the sensation of your breath.

Then let your attention go.

When your attention is not fixed on something and is let go, you open up to that space between daydreaming and concentrating.

This space is still and quiet...until things pop up.

Things will pop up.

These could be thoughts, emotions, images, or sensations.

They appear.

You observe.

You don't judge them or follow them.

They happened, and now they are done.

You return to the quiet stillness.

Just. Sit.

When another thing pops up, repeat.

They appear.

You observe.

You don't judge them or follow them.

They happened, and now they are done.

You return to the quiet stillness.

Just. Sit.

When your timer goes off, return to the external world.

The reason that thought observation meditation is so effective is because it makes you carve out time to focus on what is really happening in your monkey brain. The monkey brain chatters endlessly. All the fucking time. However, if you take the time to send your attention that way, then it doesn't know what to do. As soon as you say, "I'm listening," it starts stuttering and slowing down. Finally, it shuts up.

A yoga teacher of mine once compared this to shadow monsters. She said that in the dark, we often see things in shadows, but if we shine some light on them, the shadows go away. I am far less eloquent than she is, so I would say that it's like the grown-ups finally showed up to the department store and started leaving with their respective caffeinated toddlers. The toddlers have suddenly grown quiet, perhaps even polite. Peace is restored.

Beginning a new meditation practice isn't always easy. It can be discouraging if you find that your mind wanders often and easily. This doesn't mean you're doing it wrong! The goal isn't to be completely devoid of thoughts. The goal is to create a space where you can observe the ones that do show up without attaching to them and to do it often enough that you begin to find space between.

Starting out, you may find it hard to sit for long periods of time. It's common; don't worry about it! Try starting with short sessions. Even just three minutes every day or two can go a long way. It can also be helpful to keep notes about your experiences. Try tracking the thoughts, emotions, and sensations that come up, especially if there are recurring themes. You can also track how long you sat for, how much still space you found, and perhaps even how you felt before and after your meditation. This info can be insightful! Keeping track of it can encourage you to stick with it, even when things get tough.

Some days will be easy; others will be hard.

Once upon a time, in a land far, far away...I trained in circus arts in Beijing. A fellow named Alex was also training there, and he did some pretty incredible aerial arts.

Sometimes I would have a bad training day, and it would feel as if all the progress I had made was slipping away from me. I would get incredibly disappointed with myself, and my frustration was obvious to everyone.

Alex, however, never seemed to have bad training days. He always worked his ass off with a smile and couldn't wait to tell us about his progress after our classes. I was a little (a lot) jealous of the fact that he seemed to constantly be improving and I was taking spontaneous leaps backward.

One day, I asked Alex how he never seemed to have bad training days, and he told me that he did have them. He had them often! He just never let it get to him, because he knew that the bad days made the good ones possible. He had to put in the work on those crappy days in order to lay the foundation for the days when he kicked ass. On those bad days, he realized that even if he was struggling with something that was usually easy for him now, he could remember the time when it was completely impossible. They reminded him how far he had come.

My mind was blown. Since then, whenever I'm having a things-are-harder-than-they-should-be day, I remind myself that I have to work with the shit days in order to get the kick-ass ones. It made it a lot easier to laugh at my own mistakes and be patient with myself when I struggled.

It's important to cut yourself some slack on the days that suck. At times, you might feel that you're going backward, but you're not. The path of improvement is never direct, but you'll get there as long as you don't quit. Honor your own pace; it doesn't have to be a sprint! Just, no matter what, keep putting one foot in front of the other, even—no, *especially*—when it's hard.

At first, it might feel weird as hell. You might even feel guilty or selfish about taking time entirely for yourself to do something that looks like a whole lot of nothing from the outside. Those weirdo feelings do subside, and it gets easier. Soon it will become strange *not* to do it.

Starting a thought observation meditation practice isn't going to magically make your hair double in thickness or make a Porsche show up in your driveway. The benefits are much more subtle than that, but if you stick with it, they will be life changing. You will start thinking more efficiently and from a place of clarity. You will understand yourself better and tap into your intuition, and your monkey brain will quiet down. A meditation practice is key to becoming Zen as fuck, both inside and out.

Posture

A meditation practice will not only affect the way you think, it will also affect the way you move. People who practice regularly find that they move with more confidence and precision and that their overall posture is improved.

That might sound super outlandish at first, but just think about it! When you're having a down-in-the-dumps kind of day, how do you carry yourself? Chances are that you aren't exactly channeling your inner Beyoncé. You're not strutting around like you own the place. Nah! You're probably hunching over and dragging your heels when you walk. You might find some loose change on the ground as you avoid eye contact, staring at your shoes, but that's about the only upside. However, when you're channeling your inner badass and feeling like a motherfuckin' rock star, you're going to hold your chin high. You'll stand up straight and move with purpose. Strangers will see your body language and inherently understand that you are majestic. As. Fuck.

A couple of quick questions for you before we carry on:

* How do you generally move and carry yourself?
* What do you think this says about your state of mind?

POSTURE VS. THOUGHT EXPERIMENT

How closely are thoughts and posture related, really? Let's do a brief experiment so you can feel it out for yourself.

Think about a shitty time in your life.

You know...*that* time! How could you forget?

How did it feel?

Did it hurt? Did you feel alone?

I bet you felt like garbage.

What thoughts were running through your head?

How did you feel about yourself?

What were you telling yourself?

Think about that shitty time, remembering it all clearly.

Sit in this shit for a minute.

Let.

It.

Steep.

Notice your posture. How are you holding yourself? Notice your face, hands, shoulders, and chest. How do your muscles feel? How are you breathing?

▶ **Now try this one:**

Remember an incredible moment in your life.

Yeah, *that* time! It was fucking awesome.

How did it feel?

Did you smile? Did you feel ecstatic?

I bet you felt truly alive.

What thoughts were running through your head?

How did you feel about yourself?

What were you telling yourself?

Think about that incredible moment, remembering it all clearly.

Sit in this greatness for a minute.

Let.

It.

Steep!

Notice your posture. How are you holding yourself? Notice your face, hands, shoulders, and chest. How do your muscles feel? How are you breathing?

Now let's mix it up...

Bring your feet and knees together.

Clench your stomach muscles.

Cross your arms, and clench your fists.

Bring your shoulders forward and up.

Drop your chin, and let your chest cave in.

Speed up your breathing.

Lock this posture in, and let your mind wander.

Hold this for a couple of minutes.

Let it steep.

What was going on in your mind? What were you thinking about? What were you feeling? What kind of expression did your face make?

> **Now try this one:**
> Set your feet shoulder-width apart.
>
> Relax your abdomen.
>
> Bring your hands out to your sides, and turn your palms up.
>
> Roll your shoulders back and down.
>
> Lift your gaze upward, and let your chest open.
>
> Let your breath become deep and slow.
>
> Lock this posture in, and let your mind wander.
>
> Let it steep.

What was going on in your mind? What were you thinking about? What were you feeling? What kind of expression did your face make?

Cool, right?! In the first two exercises, we played around with how thoughts affect our posture. When you thought of an incredible moment, you held yourself differently than when you thought about a shitty memory. With this in mind, it's easy to see how a regular meditation practice can vastly change your posture!

In the last two exercises, we saw that our posture can also affect our thoughts. Yes, that thought-posture connection runs both ways! This means that by changing how we carry ourselves, we can hijack our own minds. You can use this to your advantage in your daily life or to keep your cool in stressful situations: job interviews, emotional conversations, anxious days, tax season, etc. A little bit of badass posture can go a long way!

Posture doesn't just mean how upright your spine is. Sure, the spine is the most noticeable part of it, but it's so much more than that. Your arms, shoulders, knees, and ankles count too. It's a whole body thing! When your entire body is actively engaged, then so is your mind. When you stop paying attention to what your body is doing, your thoughts have an easier time wandering away. Conversely, when your thoughts take off and get real daydreamy, your body starts making decisions without consulting you. You're more prone to bad posture and nervous twitches. It's an inner-body conspiracy. But unlike conspiracies about aliens or the Illuminati, this one you can use to your advantage.

Hands

One of the ways that this inner-body conspiracy is most obvious is in our hands. First off, let's just state the obvious. Hands are fucking weird. They're just strange spindly growths attached to the end of noodle-y arm appendages. They're wonderful, awkward gifts of evolution. Although we don't spend a lot of time actively thinking about our hands, we use them to communicate with the world around us all the time. There are people who use sign language fluently, and then there are people who "talk" with their hands (and I'm definitely one of them). This is a common trait of highly emotional and passionate people. It's as though the weight and depth of their thoughts bubble over the brims of their brains, and it all comes out in wild gestures when they talk. They (we) don't do it on purpose! It just comes naturally because of how closely posture and thought are connected.

Another example is people who bite their fingernails. Sure, they might do it intentionally sometimes because "there's just this one last piece I have to get!" But most of the time, they are completely unaware of the fact that they're cannibalizing themselves. What kind of thoughts would you guess they're having while they're habitually ripping apart their own flesh?

If you guessed "fucking chaotic," then you'd be correct.

When someone is biting or picking at their fingernails, their thoughts are not quiet. Good or bad, their brain is a whirlwind of thoughts crashing into one another. It's like a room full of stockbrokers, hyped up on cocaine and espresso, screaming and shouting over one another at an unnecessary volume. They can't even hear or finish one thought through to the end before another one starts. It's so loud that it might just register as static noise.

Aaaaaaand it's personal confession time...

I stared biting my fingernails when I was three. Doing so was a coping mechanism for me to manage my anxiety, which was a real struggle for me. My thoughts were often off on unchaperoned anxious adventures of their own. The vast majority of my anxiety was internal, so from the outside, my struggle wasn't immediately obvious. I could play it cool and look comfortable at a party. I could rock public speaking and perform on a stage. If you didn't look too closely, I appeared well adjusted enough, but if you knew what to look for, you could tell I was a mess just by looking at my hands. I regularly bit, tore, and picked them until they bled. I would rarely be conscious of it until someone pointed it out or I noticed blood on my clothes...again.

I tried almost everything imaginable to stop myself. First, I tried tough love. I asked my friends to slap me if they caught me, dipped my fingers in lemon juice every night, and painted my fingernails with nasty-tasting polish. But I learned to dodge my friends without thinking about it, developed a high pain tolerance, and developed a taste for nasty shit. When tough love didn't work, I tried the softer approach. I wore gloves as often as I could without it being creepy, gave myself fancy manicures, and did frequent deep moisturizing treatments. That didn't work either. I often caught myself gnawing on one hand while the other held the glove I had subconsciously removed. I was routinely furious with myself when, in only a couple of minutes, I had picked apart a manicure that had taken me an hour to complete. The only thing that was moderately effective was the deep moisturizing treatments, but they just turned my rough gaping wounds into soft gaping ones.

I realize that I am talking about this in past tense as though it's a thing I grew out of or magically cured myself of. I sure as fuck did not. The anxiety that comes along with something like dermatillomania (which is the fancy name for chronically and drastically destroying your own skin) isn't exactly something you get rid of. Instead, you find the tools that you need, you use the hell out of those tools, and then over time, it gets easier to manage. When shit really hits the fan, I still struggle, and sometimes I fall back on this compulsion as a crutch. I'm not perfect. But! I don't cannibalize myself daily anymore, and I think that's just dandy! So how did I make it better? The tool that finally worked for me was hijacking my mind-body connection through my posture.

In yoga, there are many different hand positions, which are classically known as mudras. A mudra is said to channel a certain energy to help achieve a specific goal or mindset. There are mudras for improving focus, getting rid of a headache, curing a cold, relieving constipation, soothing the mind, etc. You get the gist. There's a mudra for everything!

The idea that you could get such targeted and seemingly uncorrelated benefits by simply holding your hands a certain way may seem far-fetched. If you're feeling a bit skeptical here, that's okay. When I first learned about mudras, I stared blankly at my yoga teacher and half expected her to tell me how flat the Earth is. You don't need to believe that holding your hands in a certain position will help reduce pain in your ears (yes, there is a mudra for that!). But since we've already proven that our thoughts and posture are a two-way street, why wouldn't holding your hands in a particular way be capable of having an effect on your mind?

Yo. Check it.

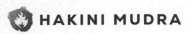

HAKINI MUDRA

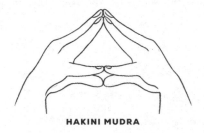

HAKINI MUDRA

You recognize this mudra, right? You've probably seen it a thousand times and never gave it much thought. I like to joke that these are "plotting hands" because they remind me of Mr. Burns from *The Simpsons*. He would always hold his hands like this when he was scheming. You have also seen real people, not just cartoon ones, do this subconsciously when they're deep in thought. You have likely done it yourself too. It makes sense because this mudra is said to help with thinking and is known for improving concentration and memory. Bonus: It's even said to help with balance!

Get your hakini mudra on by facing your palms in toward each other and forming a funky little finger tent. Leave some open space between your palms, and press your fingertips into each other to create gentle pressure.

Give 'er a go when you need to concentrate or try to remember something or are in a balancing yoga pose.

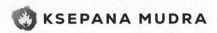

KSEPANA MUDRA

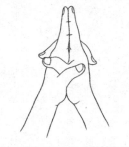

KSEPANA MUDRA FINGER GUNS

This mudra is said to be great for letting go of any Bullshit that's just not working for you. This could be stress, a crap attitude, anger, a relationship, a memory, etc. Let's be real; life throws more shit than a wild howler monkey, and sometimes it sticks with us! This mudra is said to be good for letting go of physical things too, such as sickness or pain. Note: I am not advocating this as a replacement for medical treatment. You may find ksepana mudra helpful for managing discomfort, but if you break your leg or think you have COVID-19, go see a doctor, m'kay?

Get your ksepana mudra on by touching your index fingers together and interlacing your other fingers like you're making a sweet gun with your hands. Cross your thumbs over each other, aaaaand BOOM!

Give 'er a go when you have Bullshit, of any kind, that you just gotta release.

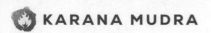

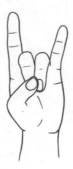

KARANA MUDRA, ROCK AND ROLL HANDS

This one is more commonly used by Buddhists, but it can be found in the yoga world too. It is classically used to "ward off evil" and to remove any obstacles that may be standing in the way of enlightenment or happiness. Its uses are very similar to the ksepana mudra, except it's more about keeping Bullshit out in the first place instead of letting it go after it's in.

Get your karana mudra on by bending your middle and ring fingers in toward your palm. Move your thumb on top of the bent fingers and press them into each other to create some light pressure. Leave your pinkie and pointer finger pointed upward and rock on!

Give 'er a go when you wanna ward off some Bullshit and feel a little more unfuckwithable.

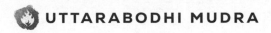

UTTARABODHI MUDRA

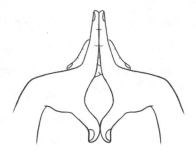

UTTARABODHI MUDRA

This is the mudra that saved me from gnawing my own hands off completely and being called "Ol' Stumpy" for the rest of my life! One day, I noticed that my hands naturally liked to rest in this position when I still and feel relaxed. It felt good, and it kept my hands out of my mouth, so I made a habit of it. Later, my yoga teacher told me it was actually a thing! She called it the "lightning rod to divinity." Classically, it is said to boost inner confidence, which helps relieve stress and anxiety. This calm and boosted state is then said to help connect to inspiration and the inner self.

Get your uttarabodhi mudra on by touching your index fingers together and interlacing your other fingers like you're making a sweet gun with your hands. Next, let your palms move away from each other as you pull your thumbs back toward yourself.

Give 'er a go when you want to feel more like a grounded and confident badass…and/or if you're chewing your freakin' hands!

Mind-Body Stillness

Stillness is something that is missing from most of our lives, which is un-fucking-fortunate, because it's powerful stuff! Mentally, emotionally, and physically, stillness has incredible benefits. When you can find stillness in your mind *and* body, these benefits get doubly awesome.

Let's explore this through yoga postures. We're going to approach these postures differently than we have been approaching the previous sequences in this book. This time around, I want you to focus on stillness, both in mind and body. See if you can summon some of that space between daydreaming and concentrating. Also, take your sweet-ass time as you make adjustments and transition between poses and hold them.

Your thoughts might start getting restless, but don't get hung up on it. Kicking yourself isn't any help! Whenever your thoughts start bouncing around, put a metaphorical pin in them, and bring your focus back to the sensation of your breath. Think about it as though you've set up an automatic mental vacation responder. Anytime something unwanted lands in your brain inbox, it receives a message right back saying "I'm not available right now, but I promise I'll get back to you later if it's actually important."

Beginning to fidget is also super normal in this stillness exercise. Our lives can be so busy and fast-paced that it's rare for us to get much stillness outside sleeping. It can be a new, weird, and sometimes frustrating experience. Kicking yourself is still not helpful. Bring your attention back to your thoughts, and calm them. It can help to count your breaths or to do some thought observation meditation.

Remember, if your body or mind becomes restless, you can hijack one by bringing stillness into the other.

Without any further fucking around, let's do this!

SLOW DOWN SEQUENCE

In this sequence, you will be holding each pose for a long time. Rather than flowing from one pose to the next, the goal is to find stillness in each one. You can start by holding each pose for two minutes. You might want to use a timer when you first start out; otherwise, you might do that thing where you can't relax because you check the time every ten seconds. Or you might do that other thing where you rush ahead to the next thing too fast because thirty seconds really does feel like two minutes when you're a fidgety person. This is not a judgment. This is my own personal experience as one super fidgety fucker!

You also might want to get some props to support you in these long holds. Yoga blocks and bolsters are great to have on hand. If you don't have yoga specific props available, then improvise by collecting whatever you have around that could be considered nap supplies. Pillows and blankets are our friends. In a pinch, scarves and sweaters can be makeshift blankets or be rolled into pillows as well.

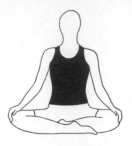

SEATED—LEGS CROSSED

Get yourself in a seated position. Make yourself extra cozy by adding any extra supports you might need. Perhaps sit on a pillow so your hips are higher than your knees. You can also try adding a blanket over your knees or placing supports under them, so your legs can be heavy without the temptation to engage them. Rest your hands on your knees and find a position where your spine is long and straight, rooting down through your tailbone and lengthening your neck. Relax your shoulders. They work so hard and they deserve a freakin' rest! Focus on your breath, perhaps even practicing your Cyclical Breath. Sit here for two minutes. Cross your legs the other way and repeat.

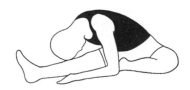

HEAD-TO-KNEE-POSE

With your fine booty on the ground, come into Head-to-Knee Pose. You can try added supports in this pose by placing them under one of your knees (or both!) You can also add something larger, like a bolster or a big pillow, between your front leg and your chest. Relax your back muscles and let your head and arms hang heavy. Keep steady in your breath and let your body melt. You may find your muscles have a mind of their own and begin to tense up. It's common and it doesn't mean you fucked up! Just be aware of it, breathe, and relax back into the pose. You may find that tossing a blanket on your back helps with this. Chill for two minutes. Repeat on the other side.

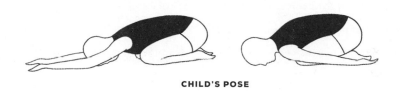

CHILD'S POSE

Child's Pose can be turned into a one person cuddle puddle pretty quickly by adding supports. It's fan-fucking-tastic. Try placing a bolster or a large pillow under your torso. You can even place something under the top end of the support to give it just enough of a lift so you can sneak your arms under and give it a hug. You can turn the cozy factor up even further by placing a blanket on your low back. Turn your head to the side, just keep breathing, and snuggle the shit out of your support for two minutes.

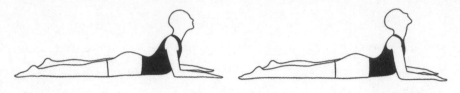

SPHINX POSE

Lying on your stomach, come into Sphinx Pose. This pose will require a little bit more work than the previous ones but you can make that work a little easier with your supports. Try placing a pillow or bolster under your chest. You can also place something more firm under your elbows. Keep a light engagement down through your elbows, shoulders, and forearms to lift and open your chest. Taking steady, deep breaths, feel your chest expand with your inhales. Feel the gentle lift of your exhale with your engaged muscles. In sphinxlike fashion, stay stoic here for two minutes.

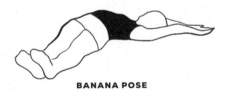

BANANA POSE

Lying on your back, bring yourself into an aPEELing Banana Pose. You can get extra comfy points by placing a support under your knees or behind your head, and tossing a blanket over yourself. Wiggle your arms and legs over to one side of your mat and find a delicious gentle side stretch. Be a banana, breathing deeply into your side body for two minutes, then repeat on the other side.

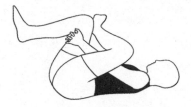

RECLINED FIGURE 4

For extra support in your Reclined Figure 4 you may want to scoot your mat up to a wall. You can rest the foot of your lower leg on the wall so the muscles can relax. With your foot on the wall, you won't have to use your hands to pull the lower leg into your body and this will make it easier to relax into the pose. You can also try placing a pillow under your head and placing a blanket over your raised feet. Since your feet will be higher than your heart, your blood won't reach them as easily, because gravity is real! Be conscious of your muscles in this pose. They will likely try to engage and tense up when you're not paying attention. Breathe, relax your shoulders, and let your hips melt into the floor. Stay here for two minutes, then repeat on the other side.

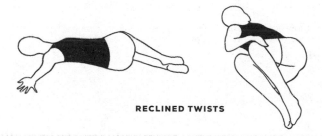

RECLINED TWISTS

Let's get twisted! There are many ways that you can use your supports in Reclined Twists and they can vary a lot from person to person. Some great options include placing a support between your knees, under the bottom knee, behind you back or under your chest. Take the time to try a couple options out to find which work best for you and your body. Found optimal coziness? Keep those badass breaths coming! Notice the sensations in your hips on your inhales and in your back on your exhales. Be aware of your muscles, especially in your hips. Melt here for two minutes and then repeat on the other side.

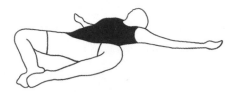

RECLINED BUTTERFLY

Come into Reclined Butterfly on your back. You can place supports under your knees, under your back, or behind your head. If you like, you can also snuggle up under a blanket. Let your arms lay open and heavy for a gentle chest opener. Keep up with your badass breaths and feel all the sensations in your chest, hips, and inner legs. Feel your chest rise on your inhales, and let your shoulders and legs melt on your exhales. Relax here for two minutes.

How did you feel after that? Zen as fuck? I hope so!

TAPPING INTO STILLNESS IS LIKE
PLUGGING DIRECTLY INTO AN
ENERGY SOURCE TO CHARGE YOUR
BATTERIES. IT CONNECTS YOUR
MIND AND BODY TO THE MOMENT,
THEN GIVES YOU THE POWER TO
NOT ONLY MOVE FORWARD...BUT
TO REALLY KICK ASS!

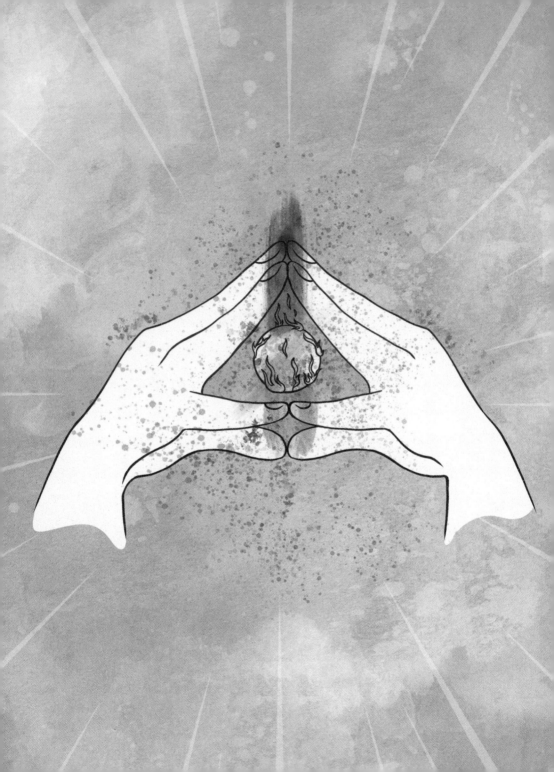

3

TRUST YOURSELF

"Instinct is a marvelous thing. It can neither be explained nor ignored."
—AGATHA CHRISTIE, *THE MYSTERIOUS AFFAIR AT STYLES*

Another badass benefit of mind-body stillness is that it gives you the ability to connect to your intuition. I know that to some of you reading this, "intuition" might sound super fluffy. That's cool; I get it. The word rubbed me the wrong way for a long time too. It seemed like it was used solely by holier-than-thou assholes, either to validate their own biases or to avoid accountability for their thoughts and actions. Yes, sometimes that *is* the case. However, intuition is a very real thing.

Before we talk about how to cultivate intuition, let's talk about what it *really* is. Intuition is knowing and understanding something without the need for words or reasoning. This is done by the subconscious parts of our brains talking to us directly, bypassing the overly rational conscious parts. The subconscious mind works much faster than the conscious one, and it speaks in a different language. Unlike the rational conscious mind, the subconscious thinks and speaks predominantly with senses and feelings. It's hard to make yourself understood by someone who barely shares a language with you, so it's no wonder we rarely hear from our intuition. Our conscious brains keep fucking up the messages!

Intuition isn't a supernatural power that allows you to see around corners or predict the future. Yet in a way, intuition is like a superpower, just not the kind that they bother making comics about. So if it doesn't mean being able to see with X-ray eyes or some shit, what is so super about intuition?

Tapping into your intuition allows you to connect with your true wisdom. That "gut feeling" or "hunch" that you get when your intuition pipes up is your subconscious trying to help you out. The subconscious knows its stuff. It knows you better than you know yourself. When you learn how to hear it properly, things just become *easier.* It will always do its best to prepare you for what is ahead by giving you the insights or nudges that you need. Developing your intuition is hugely self-empowering, and it's an important tool for a badass to have. Ignoring it completely and expecting logic to do *all* the thinking can leave a person stuck in a dead end, tired and frustrated.

But you can't trust all your thoughts to your intuition either! Whether we're aware of them or not, we develop biases throughout our lives. All the experiences we have in life give our brains data. This data then gets sorted, and our brains pick it apart, comparing it to previous data and searching for patterns in order to make sense of the world. These patterns can be simple and clear, like developing a fear of driving after being in a car accident. But they can also be subtle.

Psychology recognizes several different types of biases that can affect our thoughts, beliefs, decisions, and actions. A confirmation bias encourages us to seek and accept information that validates our preconceptions. A gender bias can make us subconsciously associate men with CEO positions or be surprised if they work as a maid. An in-group bias makes us more likely to favor people we see as already being part of our groups, like friends, family, or those who look like us. If left unchecked, our biases can take over, drawing conclusions on their own and then passing them off to us as reality. Biases aren't inherently evil, but they can be dangerous if not recognized. They can perpetuate garbage social issues like racism, sexism, and classism. They can also turn us into those holier-than-thou assholes who think they're just so "in tune with everything" that all their biases are superior intuition. That sure sounds like a self-serving bias, doesn't it?

Although at first glance, they might seem impossible to blend, like oil and vinegar, logic and intuition support each other beautifully. When they are in a healthy balance, things get (cue the confetti)...*freakin' magical!*

So if it's so bloody magical, why doesn't everyone just tap into their intuition?

Because societal expectations. Just like we've been led into the busy trap, we've also been told there is one way to be smart—being book smart. It's so widely accepted as the only meaningful form of intelligence that we are often led to believe that other forms aren't important or valid. This conventional type of intelligence places importance on the logical brain alone, so many people slowly push their intuition away, grow distrustful of it, or flat out reject it. If you don't flex those intuition muscles, they get weak and begin to atrophy. But not to worry. With time and practice, these muscles can regain their strength and grow as strong as a young Arnold Schwarzenegger!

A great way to start is by doing the things we've already talked about in this book. Clearing out the brain shit so you can truly hear yourself think will allow your monkey brain to shut up long enough for you to hear what your intuition is saying. Learning how to be still, in mind and body, will strengthen your mind-body connection and open up the channel for the two to talk to each other. I'm sure they have some catching up to do. The next step is to work on your intuition directly.

There are said to be several different kinds of intuition. Some sources will tell you about being able to foretell the future, connect to your past lives, or hear truths from a different dimension. That's not my jam. I'm not discounting it completely, but it's not my field of expertise or interest. The intuition I want to talk about is easily accessible and universally applicable in day-to-day life. Let's talk about intuitive movement.

Intuitive Movement

Intuitive movement is a combination of intuition, creativity, and improvisation. It's essentially a movement-based meditation that takes your head out of the equation and lets your body do all the thinking. It lets your body move in the ways that it needs instead of the ways that it has become accustomed to. This can help keep your on-mat practice playful and engaging while strengthening the hell out of your mind-body connection. That connection goes a long way in being able to understand and feel the mechanics and needs of your body. Overall, an intuitive movement practice is great for boosting creativity, coordination, and confidence. These badass benefits follow you off the mat as well. And it's fun!

INTUITIVE WARM-UP

Before we dive into the sequence, let's do a short warm-up. This is designed to help you listen more closely to what your body wants to do intuitively instead of what your brain thinks the body "should" do. All we're really doing is standing up, sitting on the floor, and then standing back up again. When we do this, our brains kick in and take us from point A to point B in the way they always do. Instead, we're going to take our sweet time, focus on the breath, and let the body do the thinking. Try to take a minimum of thirty seconds for each direction. If it helps, set a timer!

> **Melting Down:** Begin in a strong standing position. From here, focus on your breath, and relax your muscles. Your neck may hang, your knees can bend, and your arms might feel heavy. Let your body gradually lower to the floor, letting gravity do that thing it does, as you move at the pace of a stoned sloth. Allow your body to melt and move in whichever way feels good. Eventually, you'll find yourself in a relaxed seated position on the floor.

Building Up: From this seated position, you're going to (oh so slowly) rise back up to a standing position. Again, focus on the breath. If it helps, imagine that your breath is gradually filling you up like an inflatable bouncy castle. In the beginning, you're relaxed and compact. Then you slowly inflate, expand, and become taller. Start stacking your body in whichever way feels right, and eventually build yourself back up to a strong standing position.

You need foundational tools to build a strong yoga practice...or to build anything, really. Following direction, learning technique, and giving fucks about doing it right are necessary to acquire those tools. However, when it comes to an intuitive movement practice, "right" is going to get you nowhere. If you follow the rules all the time, like an overly keen superstar pupil waiting for a cookie, then you cheat yourself out of an ocean of possibilities. Sorry, friend, the cookies are a lie. So when it comes to an intuitive movement practice, the number one thing to keep in mind is simply this...

FUCK THE RULES!

We look (way too often) to external sources for answers to our internal questions or some measure of "rightness," because it's easy. It's harder to find the answers in ourselves, and it can be even harder to trust them. Let your intuition take the wheel from time to time. It will bring a lot of creativity and power into your yoga practice. Say it with me now...

FUCK THE RULES!

 INTUITIVE SEQUENCES

In this sequence, we're going to do things a little differently. Rather than give you exact directions, I am going to give you the rough framework of a sequence. You'll get suggestions here and there, but the goal is to let your own body do the instructing. Follow your intuition. Hold the poses as long as you like, modify what you want, and add anything you need.

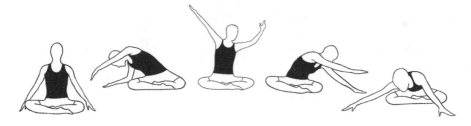

Begin in a natural seated position and take your hands to wherever feels comfortable. Check in with your body. Warm, cold, relaxed, stiff... Are any areas feeling noteworthy sensations? Make whatever adjustments that feel right and breathe here. When you're ready, let's start to play! Place your hands on the mat, tracing them in any direction you like. Let your body move, following your hands.

Trust Yourself

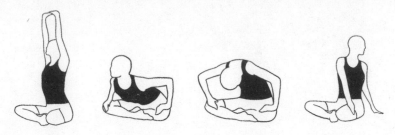

While you're still in this seated position, let's get that spine moving! You can explore lengthening, scooping, twisting, and arching. Trust yourself and trust your body to lead you in the ways that it craves.

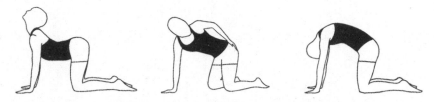

Coming up onto all fours, keep experimenting with that spinal movement. Like any good scientist, you can add new variables like lifting limbs or moving your gaze in different directions.

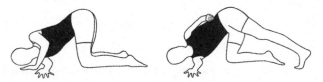

From this tabletop position on all fours, thread one arm under your chest and lower your head to the mat. Start moving around while keeping your bottom shoulder in place. You can try shifting your weight back and forth or side to side. You can turn your chest toward the mat or open it up to the wall. Take note of how the sensations in your body change as you explore different corners of this pose.

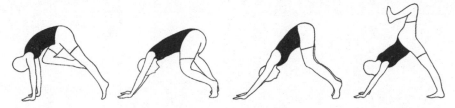

Come back up onto all fours, then while keeping your hands on the mat, lift your hips up high. Get comfortable here, taking deep breaths and making any adjustments that feel right to you. Once you've found a strong home base in this pose, begin fucking with it. Shift your weight back and forth between your hands and feet. Try twisting your body, raising and lowering your hips, moving your neck and lifting limbs. Get curious! Stay steady in your breath and let your body lead.

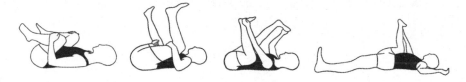

Make your way down to the mat and lay on your back. Start by hugging your knees into your chest. Ground yourself here, feeling how the sensation of your breath ripples through your body as it comes and goes. Now...fuck around some more! How does your body want to move here? Does it want to stay still or rock side to side? Does it feel good to bend or straighten your legs?

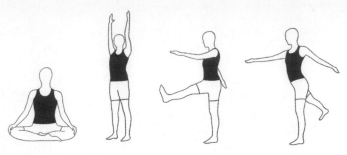

Begin to bring yourself into a seated position. Don't just "sit up." Fuck that. Listen to your body and let it lead the way. Pause in this seated position to check in with dat bod and breath. Then move on, making your way into a standing position. Again, pause. Check in. Notice the way your weight comes into your feet and how they connect you to the mat. When you're ready, shift your weight into one foot and let the other float off the ground. Let your raised foot gently sway and then gradually begin to swing. Allow your body to move, naturally counterbalancing the weight of the swinging leg. Once you're satisfied, repeat on the other side.

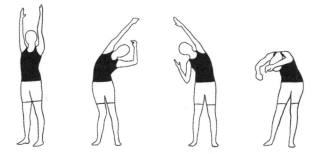

Float your hands up high overhead, letting your torso sway, bend, and twist in any way that feels right. Notice how your arms, neck, and knees intuitively follow. Breathe, observe how it feeds into this movement, letting your body move you through fantastic nameless shapes.

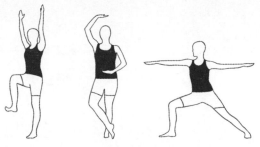

Shift your weight into one foot and let the other lift off the mat. Experiment with your lifted leg, perhaps lifting it high or crossing it over your standing leg. When you move your leg, how does your core move? How do your arms move to help you balance? Take some badass breaths here, feeling how your body adjusts to balance and support you. When you're ready, step your lifted foot back and observe how the rest of you instinctively moves to make this happen.

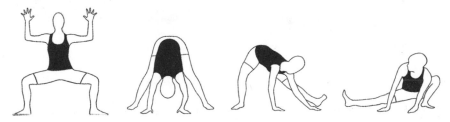

Ever so slightly lifting your heels, come up onto the balls of your feet and turn your body to the open side of your mat. Inhale, bringing your hands up overhead. Exhale, following your body's instincts as you slowly let your torso melt down and bring your hands onto the mat. Hang heavy here for a moment and check in. How does your body want to move here? Listen to your instincts and fuck around.

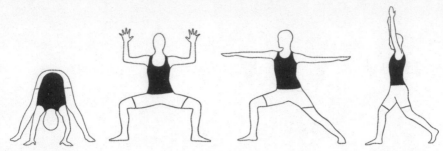

From this folded position, center your weight between your feet and take a slight bend in your legs. Gradually "un-melt," building yourself upright again. Stay steady in your breath and be aware of your how body chooses to move. Once you've come all the way up, keep your feet in place as you lift your heels and begin rotating back to the front of your mat.

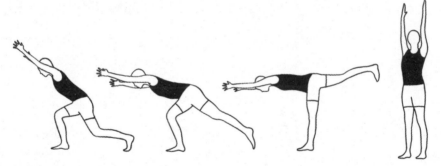

Take a slight bend in your knees and start to send your weight forward, gradually taking your weight into your front foot. Trust yourself and breathe as you continue to move forward, slowly lifting your back foot off of your mat and straightening your front leg back behind you. Don't let your head get in the way by micromanaging yourself! Instead, get curious! Watch how your body adjusts and moves to balance itself. Stay in this balance for a little and feel it out. Once you're satisfied, bring your back leg forward and step into a standing position. In any way that feels good, give yourself a "fuck yeah!"

Feels great, right? At first, it might feel kind of strange, and perhaps like you have no idea WTF is really going on with your body. I like to call this "awkward baby giraffe" syndrome. However, once you get a feel for it, it opens an endless playground of possibilities. Getting in the habit of breaking the rules and trusting your body will help you get there.

Structure is great! Still, too much of a good thing turns into a bad thing. Relying too heavily on structure can minimize your creativity, cut you off from your Badass Self, and make you feel like you're stuck in a rut. Trusting ourselves and exploring intuitively is such a simple yet uncommon solution, in life and on the yoga mat! However, the fact that it's simple doesn't mean that it's easy. It can take a lot of pep-talking and courage to stray from the safety, familiarity, and approval that structure provides. Even if it's exploring new movement in your own body, venturing into unknown territory can be scary. It feels a lot like stepping out of line, and since we were children, we've been told that we're *not even supposed to color outside the lines!*

Fuck that.

When you create space for your intuition to guide your body, it gets more accustomed to speaking up, and you get better at listening. Your intuition is no dummy. Let it be a trusted advisor as you make your own rules in your yoga practice and on your mat. Let yourself move in new, weird, and wonderful ways. While you're at it, color outside the lines if it makes you happy! In fact, I'm going to encourage you to take that very literally in a minute. But first, let's circle back to meditation and explore more corners of stillness.

Meditation Techniques

So far, we've touched on a couple of different kinds of meditation. We talked about thought observation and dabbled in a few ways that include movement. But meditation has many other forms too! Anything that puts you into a badass "flow state" can be called meditative. People often find this state through things like walking, juggling, singing, dancing, or painting. Chances are that at some point in your life, you've had one of these experiences while doing an activity you enjoy, even if you didn't call it meditative at the time.

Yoga has many different traditional forms of mediation. We're going to cover the basics and explore some of them now. I'll also give you examples of how you might tweak them to make them work for you.

Japa Meditation

Japa is the practice of repeating one of the many names of God, or a mantra, over and over. The idea is that by repeating a mantra, or a name of God, you are protecting your mind. As we already know, the monkey brain is a chatterbox that, when left to its own devices, is kind of an asshole. By repeating something over and over, in our heads or out loud, we are giving it something to fix its attention on. This keeps the mind focused instead of getting swept away in chaos. This can help "purify" the mind and keep Bullshit from entering.

The most simple mantra and the one that you've definitely heard before is "om." They get longer and fancier from there. Seriously. Traditional yoga never skimps on details! There are countless traditional mantras for different goals and intentions.

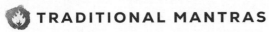

TRADITIONAL MANTRAS

Here are a couple of examples of traditional mantras.

Om Ham So Ham
As is God, so am I.

Om Gum Ganapatayei Namaha
Remove obstacles and bestow wisdom.

Om Apadamapa Hataram Dataram Sarva Sampadam Loka Bhi Ramam
Sri Ramam Bhuyo Namam-Yaham
O compassionate Rama. Please send your healing energy right here to the Earth, to the Earth. Salutations.

Unless you know Sanskrit or are hard-core enough to learn it, it might feel strange to use these traditional mantras. If you don't know the words, it can feel really robotic or forced. Or maybe you'll feel like a character on an episode of *Buffy the Vampire Slayer*. You know, the poor soul who accidentally reads a spell from a sacred tome and then gets possessed or unleashes a demon or starts bleeding from their eyes or something.

Some people prefer to stick to tradition. If that's you, kudos! Do your thing. However, many people end up shying away from this practice completely because it just doesn't fit. If it doesn't fit and it doesn't feel good, you're probably not going to use it, and that defeats the purpose entirely! Then it's like a fondue kit. Great in theory, but in reality, it just collects dust and guilty feelings. If you can adjust and personalize aspects of a practice in a way that means you will actually use it, do so. Nobody needs another fondue kit. If a mantra doesn't feel right for you, try out affirmations.

Affirmations

The concept of affirmations used to really make me roll my eyes. It sounded like some crap that cubicle workers learned about in office-wide, mandatory self-esteem-building workshops. Or like the tacky inspirational quotes that you find on posters, which somehow always look like they're from the 1980s despite being brand-new and almost exclusively end up in those office spaces. But that was back when I was cannibalizing my own hands and battling internal demons on a daily basis. I've come around since then! Affirmations are powerful shit. They can be used in a similar way to mantras. They don't sound as pretty as traditional Sanskrit, but they still do the job of giving your chatterbox brain something awesome to fix its attention on.

Affirmations can be customized for your needs. If you're feeling nervous about something, you could repeat to yourself, "I am calm. I am collected. I am Zen as fuck." It might sound like you're lying to yourself at first, but things will begin to shift. Repetition is key! Every time you repeat them, these words become stronger in your mind. This is how ancient words became sacred. Through repetition and the passing of time, the meaning of these words soaks in. They begin to carry personal weight and power. Eventually, what started off as nonsense, silly words becomes real and unfuckwithable.

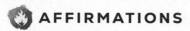

AFFIRMATIONS

Here are some affirmations I love.

I am open to receive, to learn, to create.
Useful when feeling closed off, creatively stuck, or when learning new things.

I am strong. I am confident. I am a badass.
Helpful for tackling intimidating challenges and when you're feeling not so unfuckwithable.

I will do no harm. I will take no shit.
A reminder about balance and to be gentle but firm.

I embrace the past with courage and joy. I embrace this moment with courage and joy. I embrace the future with courage and joy.
Useful for feelings of anxiety, fear, or helplessness. Helpful when needing self-acceptance, forgiveness, and a feeling of contentment in the present (this one has saved my ass more than I care to admit!).

You might want to use some extra tools to help you focus with this. Again, repetition is important in this practice! If you're getting distracted by shiny things and uninvited thoughts, it's hard to get many repetitions in. Attention spans are generally painfully short and delicate, so some extra assistance can go a long way. There are many tools to help hold concentration, both traditional and nontraditional.

Japa Mala

This is when japa is paired with *mala* beads. The beads help to count how many times you've repeated the words you've chosen. They can also keep your mind from wandering by adding a physical object to focus on into the equation. These beads are used in both Hindu and Buddhist practices. Similar tools are often used by other groups, such as the Catholic rosary or Islamic prayer beads. Although the specifics of how to use the tools are different for each group, the general idea is mostly the same across the board.

Traditional yogis often use mala beads. Malas have 108 beads plus an extra funky one, called the *meru*, that connects the whole thing. The beads are meant to lie over the middle finger and be held in the right hand above the heart. The index finger is never supposed to touch the mala, because it is said to be associated with the ego. For each time you say your mantra, you pull one bead toward you with your thumb. Once you get all the way around the string, you flip it over and go the other way without crossing over the meru. When you get to the meru, you stop to reflect and give thanks to those who have guided you with their teachings. Switching directions symbolizes being free from the cycles of reincarnation and karma.

Tradition and ritual go hand in hand to form customs that have been performed by people for ages. A practice with such rich history and deep roots can be comforting and profoundly meaningful for many people. Others may find that this can make the idea of taking part in it seem strange or intimidating. If the idea using traditional mala beads seems like the wrong fit for you, you might try an alternative tool.

Regular-Old-Whatever Beads

If the tradition of the mala beads doesn't feel comfortable for you, you might like some regular-old-whatever beads. This is not a technical term. I just made it up. All the same, you can use a necklace or a bracelet and call it whatever you like. You just need something with beads. You can pair the beads with a mantra or try out an affirmation instead. Just like with the mala, the idea is to count a bead with each repetition. You don't need to worry about how many times you repeat it. You don't need to worry about how you hold it. You just choose what you want to remind yourself of, grab your beads, and go! This can be done anywhere. I've done this walking, backstage fighting nerves at a show, in the middle of a workday at my desk, under the table at a restaurant, etc. It's easy, it's portable, and it's powerful.

SHOUT IT FROM THE ROOFTOPS! OR DON'T

There are lots of options to choose from!

A mantra or an affirmation.

Mala beads, regular-old-whatever beads, or no beads.

Now you get to decide how loud you want to be about it.

You can say your repetitions out loud.

You can whisper them to yourself.

Or you can just repeat them in your head!

Out loud can help with concentration.

Repeating it in your head is traditionally said to be the most powerful. Whispering is a solid middle ground between the two.

As always: do what feels good!

There's still one more way that you can repeat your mantra or affirmation. It's good to explore all the options to find out which works best for you, right? Plus, who knows? Maybe beads just aren't for you because you have a legitimate phobia of spherical objects. It's a thing, sfairesphobia. Honestly, I didn't make that up.

Likhita Japa

Instead of using beads or repeating a mantra at various decibels, *likhita japa* uses the act of writing. Traditionally, this is done using a mantra, but by now, you're probably well aware that this is a "choose your own adventure" kind of book. If you prefer to use an affirmation, go for it. You can write your mantra or affirmation repeatedly across a piece of paper or, if you're feeling especially artsy, create designs with the words.

Written Meditation

Whatever you decide to write, there are many ways to write it.

You can choose black and white or introduce some color.

You can write in lines or get c r e a t i v e.

The choice is yours.

I chose to make an abstract picture out of "Zen as fuck!" To begin, I laid down some lines and circles on a blank piece of paper to create different sections. Then I filled each section in by writing my affirmation. I created some extra texture by writing in different ways.

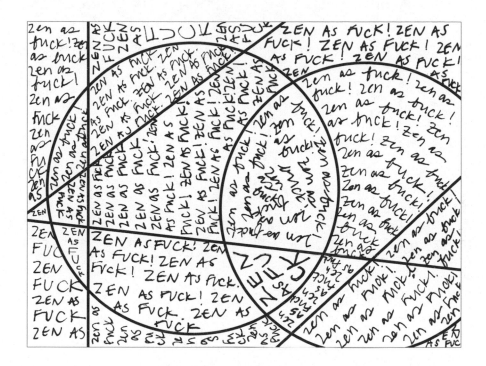

You make the rules for your practice, so you can create your own template however you like. But you gotta start somewhere, right? Here is the template I used. Grab something to write with, and give it a try! Before you begin, choose what you're going to write. If you don't have something in mind, revisit the section on affirmations and mantras for some inspiration.

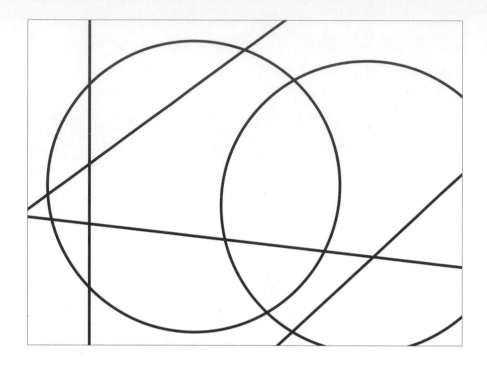

Chill Out and Color Some Shit

Maybe writing the same thing over and over isn't your thing. If not, let's try another adjustment. Instead of writing the words, why not color the words? Or even just color, for that matter? After all, coloring books don't have to just be for kids. Who makes the rules about who can color in a book? Who says which books you're allowed to color in and which ones you can't? Why couldn't this book about Rage Yoga *also* be a coloring book? Fuck it.

The act of coloring can be very soothing, with or without the addition of words. It can simply be an easy and accessible way to put yourself into a meditative state. Earlier, I told you to break the rules and color outside the lines if it made you happy. So now is your chance! Grab something to color with, throw on some good music, and let the chill times roll.

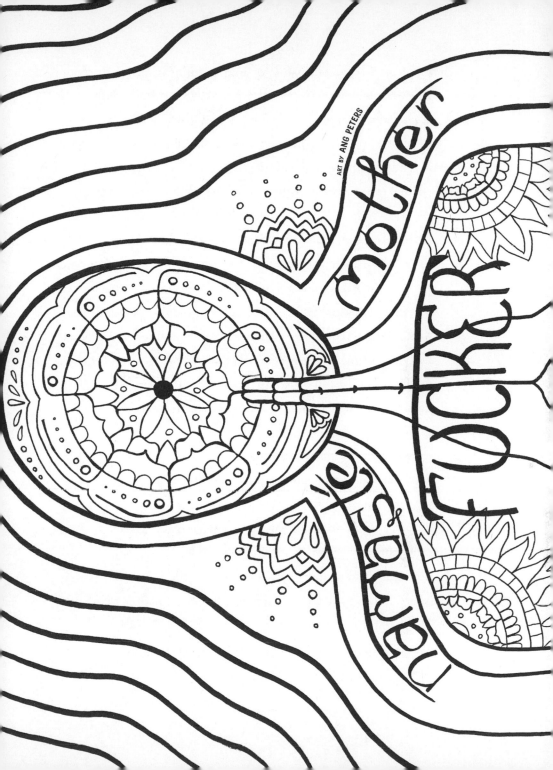

ART BY ANG PETERS

There are many different paths to finding stillness, inside and out. We've talked about taking a shit with the mind, explored the mind-body connection, played with intuitive movement, and learned about both traditional and nontraditional meditations. We broke the rules, we colored shit, and we had a damn good time doing it!

With all that ground covered, three big things should be clear by now:

1. There are a ton of different forms of meditation. No one is right or wrong or better or worse than another. Some work for some people, and others don't. The key is always to find what works and then do more of that. Also, keep in mind that you don't have to stick to just one! If you enjoy a couple of different methods, that's awesome. You may also find that your preferences change over time, and it can be helpful to switch it up once in a while. A diversified practice can help keep it fresh and keep you on track to optimal badassery.

2. Classical yogic rituals and traditions have a lot to teach us. They have long and rich histories that should be respected. However, if your current views and values don't line up with them in a way that feels genuine, these rules and rituals could keep you from practicing altogether. It's important to learn about the traditions and understand where the rituals come from, and it's also important to build a practice that feels good to you. Otherwise, you might not do it at all!

3. There is overwhelming power in stillness. It helps us relieve stress, improve mental clarity, and feel better in our bodies.

It allows us to dive down the paths of self-discovery and self-love and to tap into our intuitive inner Badass Selves. Be still and listen to yourself. You're worth listening to. YOU ARE A BADASS!

Can I get a "Fuck yeah!"?

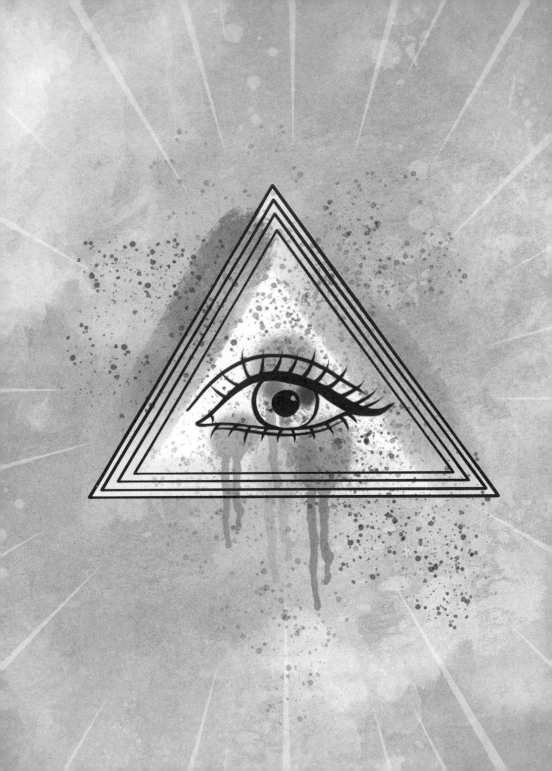

BE
UNAPOLOGETICALLY
AWESOME

"Your fear of looking stupid
is holding you back."
—RUPAUL

Hey, you.

Yes, you.

You are fucking awesome!

Has anyone told you that lately? Have you told yourself?

**WHEN WAS THE LAST TIME
YOU TOLD SOMEONE ELSE
THAT YOU'RE AWESOME?**

That's a thing you can do! You don't need anyone's permission, but if you want it, you have mine. Now maybe you're asking yourself what kind of person just up and tells other people that they're awesome. Maybe you're picturing someone who is self-obsessed, some douchebag bro, or a person who is desperately trying to cover up their own self-loathing. We've all met that person, and their awesomeness is debatable. But that's not what we're talking about here. We're talking about being unapologetically (and authentically) awesome.

Being unapologetically awesome doesn't mean puffing out your chest like an egotistical jerk and making hollow claims of greatness. It means knowing your Badass Self, loving the fuck out of it, and letting it shine... flaws and all!

Being unapologetically awesome should be the norm, but it's far from it. All our lives, we have been receiving conflicting messages about how we should feel about ourselves and how we should display that. You should value your smarts, but don't answer right away or you're a know-it-all. You should take pride in your talents, but don't display them too loudly or you're a show-off. You should love yourself, but showing it makes you a cocky asshole. In fact, openly accepting and agreeing when someone compliments you makes you an even bigger cocky asshole. So what're you supposed to do? Hide away the things that you love about yourself so no one knows you feel good about them? Awkwardly avoid eye contact when other people voice their appreciation for things you feel good about?

We get told over and over again to "be yourself," that "confidence is key," and to "live your best life." But at the same time, we're being told that we're "too much," and we should really just "tone it down." It's hard to do all those things at once! So we often settle for toning it down, hiding away the qualities that best define our experience and make us unique. Essentially, we sacrifice our awesomeness in exchange for the basic comfort of the social norm. Why is that? What do the people around us have to gain by our pretending to be less than our full potential?

Social Scripts and Conditioning

At the risk of sounding like a conspiracy theorist, I believe that a large amount of the problem is rooted in the interest of capitalism. Sheep who have been taught to believe that they are not awesome are much more likely to spend money on the things that are advertised to make them more awesome. Still, these conflicting messages aren't solely brought to us by corporations. These messages are also often brought to us by the people around us, sometimes by those who care for us the most.

When people in my local community of Calgary, Alberta, asked about regular classes, I wanted to make that happen! I knew we were onto something really cool, but I needed the right space to make it happen. It needed to be Dickens Pub. With diverse events, an inclusive and laid-back atmosphere, and the coolest local owners, it had everything I wanted!

To make this dream a reality, I had to ask. This included setting up an appointment with the owners to pitch the idea. But...what if they said no? What if they thought I was a lunatic and tore my idea to shreds? Even worse, what if they said yes and it flopped?! It would be humiliating. These were people who ran my favorite venue and who had deep roots in a community that I was new to. There were so many possible outcomes, and a lot of them ended with me looking like a freakin' idiot. But I had to try.

I asked a friend if he would go to the meeting with me. I was nervous and thought his support would help. I told him about the past workshops and how I wanted to create classes. I bribed him with a pint of beer, and he said he would come. When we were finally at Dickens, waiting for the meeting with pints in hand, his tune changed.

Perhaps the idea was just bizarre enough that the full details got fuzzy for him. Maybe he remembered the yoga part but subconsciously substituted the bar for a studio. Or maybe he remembered the Dickens Pub part but subconsciously substituted the Rage Yoga classes for hosting a circus event. I don't know what exactly happened or how. All I know for sure is that my friend forgot why we were there, and he looked real freaked out when I reminded him.

"Do you think that's a good idea? I mean, yoga is usually done in a studio. I don't know if something like that could happen in a place like this."

I instantly flipped from determined to terrified. I excused myself to the bathroom to deal with my sudden panic. I was minutes away from making an obscure proposal to people I admired, and my supportive friend had accidentally just done a roundhouse kick on the shaky foundation of my confidence. He was right. Yoga was usually done in a studio, and while I thought it had some badass potential, I was not positive it was a "good idea."

I breathed in the Good Shit. I exhaled the Bullshit. I went back to the table, and I went through with the meeting.

And lo and behold, the meeting went well! Dickens Pub was where the first official classes happened and where the whole thing took off. If I had listened to my friend, then none of it would have ever happened, and you wouldn't be reading this book. Still, I'm not upset about what my friend said. Sure, the timing was shit, but I get it. He really cared about me, and I was doing something that wasn't scripted. I was loudly trying to make something different happen, and doing so meant I was opening myself up to criticism and failure. He wasn't trying to hurt me; he was trying to keep me safe.

Our truest selves can be loud, controversial, and different. Our goals and aspirations, the things that really fulfill us, aren't always shared or understood. Letting those colorful qualities shine or pursuing things that are different is risky stuff. The outcomes are unpredictable, and that freaks people out. Parents, friends, lovers, relatives, teachers—the people who care for us most are the ones who are most invested in keeping us safe and happy. They just don't always share the same definition of "safe and happy" or know how best to protect us. It can lead to an oh-so-confusing (and sometimes hurtful) cocktail of conflicting messages and unhelpful support.

Do any of these sound familiar?

* You're being too much.
* You should dress more like this.
* Maybe you should get this job instead.
* Just be happy.
* I don't think you can handle that.

The ones we love don't pass these messages on because they're trying to keep us down or make money off us. They see all our strength, capabilities, and the things that make us awesome. They want us to see those things in ourselves too. But they also don't want us to stray too far from convention because they don't want to see us hurt. So for better or for worse, they pass these messages along out of a sense of protection.*

These messages have been handed down for generations and shared so widely that they have become a social norm. This norm is somewhat of a play script, and just like in the theater, we expect people to play their roles. These scripts have existed for such a long time that, whether we are aware of it or not, we believe their structure and predictability will keep us safe. So we keep buying into them and passing them along. This social conditioning encourages many people to read roles and lead lives that they don't actually want. The outcome is often that people feel "safe" but rarely feel genuinely happy. It's hard to find a sense of happiness or fulfillment in a structure that is entirely dependent on external approval.

One of the most important laws of the script is that our validity and

---

* Note: even overbearing and controlling tendencies often come out of a misguided sense of protection!

worth is decided by others. This can lead to a lot of time spent waiting on other people to tell us what we are. Smart, funny, good-looking, creative, or whatever. We don't need someone else's approval in order to see these things in ourselves, but we often hold out for it anyhow. It's a garbage habit, and can we take a second to acknowledge how absurd it is? We're supposed to wait for approval to be awesome, but our societal conditioning has already made it hard to just take a fucking compliment?! You're damned if you and damned if you don't. The duality of it all can give you a migraine.

Duality and Illusion

Like all philosophy, there are many branches of yogic philosophy, with varying schools of thought that were inspired by different philosophers or sages. Patanjali was one of these sages. Patanjali's classical yoga views say that the world is full of duality because matter and consciousness are two different things. This means the ever-changing material world that we know, which is made of matter, keeps us from understanding the deeper reality and the truth of consciousness. Patanjali said that the only way we can be free from duality is to overcome this separation of matter and consciousness by becoming one with God through yoga. This is because the only eternal and unchanging thing, the only real truth, is God.

Another branch of yogic thinking, the Advaita Vedanta school, says consciousness and matter are not separate. Still, even though they are not separate, this does not mean that we're free from duality. This school says that we can't see the deeper truth of reality because the world is full of illusions, otherwise known as *maya*. Maya is often directly translated as "illusion," but it has a much deeper meaning that's worthy of an essay. For now, we can boil it down to the endless and inescapable contradictions and cycles of life. The only way to see through the illusions or maya and then to be free of them is to become enlightened through yoga.

I think it's easy to see a pattern here. The world is full of a lot of Bullshit. To see through it, you have to take yourself off autopilot and wake the fuck up. You have to think for yourself, look inward, and build a healthy connection to that "something greater," whatever that means for you! Can you start by recognizing the illusions built into your social conditioning and choose to free yourself from them? Can you decide who you are for/by yourself and embody the hell out of that without waiting for the permission of others? Hell yeah, you can!

Once upon a time, there was a young person named Lindsay. They were awkward as hell. How do I know? C'mon, it was me. I would fucking know.

I liked funky hats. I still do! When I was in my early twenties, I went through a bowler hat phase. It was a whole thing. One summer day, I found a funky new one in a dollar store. It wasn't too shabby! It was inexpensive and fun. Most importantly, I felt good in it. I was in a convenience store when a kind stranger noticed it. They said, quite simply, "I like your hat."

That should have been an easy social exchange, right? It's a fucking compliment. Responding isn't exactly rocket surgery. Perhaps something simple like "thank you" would have been appropriate. Or maybe I could have gotten a bit fancy and said something like "Thanks. It's new, and it makes me feel dapper." Instead, I said this:

"Yeah? It's cheap, but it's not bad. I got it for, like, $3."

This person wasn't having it. Their tone quickly went from friendly and engaging to very much the opposite.

"I didn't ask how much it cost," they said, irritated, rolling their eyes and dismissing me. "I just thought you should know it looked nice."

I'm not going to lie to you, because a Catholic child once told me that lying burns a hole in your soul, and it was really unsettling. I left that interaction feeling pissed off at them. At the time, as far as I was concerned, I had accepted their compliment, and suddenly they turned into a dick about it. WTF?

It's funny how interactions like this can stick with you. It's not because they're grand or elaborate. Quite the opposite! They stick with you the way a sliver does. They get under your skin and stay there. Then you spend a bunch of time trying to figure out what the cause of the discomfort is, and you're unsure if there really is one at all. But eventually, it works its way to the surface, and you can see what caused the irritation.

Although it took a while, I finally worked out why the hat compliment conundrum was so uncomfortable. They were right. I had responded to their compliment by downplaying the awesomeness of the hat, and by doing so, I had casually downplayed my own awesomeness. In most social interactions, this is normal, so to me, their reaction was the strange one. They pointed out the fact that I was unable to genuinely take the compliment. It was like nails on a chalk-board. It was something you weren't supposed to do.

This wasn't the first or the last time I did this. Hell, we've all done it! In this big, busy world, this stuff may seem small, but these tiny sliver-like moments are symptoms of a bigger problem. When we habitually downplay our awesomeness, we lower the self-esteem baseline for ourselves. We also lower it for the people around us by normalizing this behavior. Don't read the social script just to play a role that is less than who you are. You're amazing. Take the compliment. I dare you.

BADASS HOMEWORK: SPREAD THE GOOD SHIT

Assignment 1: Give Compliments

See someone working hard and killing it? Tell them! Notice qualities in someone that you admire? Let them know! Eat something exceptional? Praise the cook! Hand out compliments readily when they are well deserved and when you mean them.

Assignment 2: Receive Compliments

The next time someone gives you a compliment, check in to see what your natural go-to reaction is. If you catch yourself downplaying or shying away from the compliment, then ask yourself why that is. Maybe you don't feel it's deserved. Maybe it draws attention to something that you feel is imperfect or incomplete. Or maybe, just maybe, you're exchanging your awesomeness for the basic comfort of a social norm. You are worthy, you majestic badass! Take the damn compliment.

Assignment 3: Don't Wait to Be Awesome

Don't wait for other people's permission to like who you are or what you've done. Give yourself validation instead of seeking it from others. Your homework here is to tell at least two people about something you're proud of. These can be qualities about yourself or things you've done. It could even be as simple as "I just rocked that parallel parking job!"

Don't be afraid to take joy in who you are or in your accomplishments. There is a big difference between sharing the joy they bring you and just shoving them in someone else's face until they give you a cookie. As long as that joy is a shared experience and you can comfortably share in the joy of others without making it about you, you're not being an egotistical cock knob. You're allowed to be proud of who you are and what you do.

Perceiving Our Reality in Three Layers

Part of the reason we have a hard time seeing through Bullshit is because the method in which we perceive it is flawed. When we collect information from our senses, we process it in several layers. This forms our experience, allowing us to perceive the world and create our personal reality. Yogic philosophy says this process happens in three layers.

1. The mind (*manas*)

2. The intellect (*buddhi*)

3. The ego (*ahamkara*)

The first part, the mind or *manas*, is the part that gathers the information from our senses. It sees, hears, smells, feels, and tastes. The second part, the intellect or *buddhi*, differentiates and makes sense of the information gathered from the first layer. It sees brown, smells cinnamon, feels heat, and tastes sweetness. It says, "This is pie." The third layer, the ego or *ahamkara*, goes "Hell yeah! I fucking love pie! This is pretty good, but my mom's apple pie is definitely better. I'll fight anyone who says otherwise."

Seriously. People get very defensive about their family's baking.

Pie and yogic philosophy have something in common here. When it comes to pie, people have varying understandings of what makes it good. Your tastes might be different from mine, but outside our personal preferences, pie is still pie. When it comes to the yogic understanding of how we perceive reality, the number of layers and exact terms used to describe the process change depending on who you talk to. Although there are differences found in varying schools of thought, the general theory is still the same. Basically, we collect unbiased and real information in the mind through our senses. Next, the intellect makes sense of that information by labeling and sorting it. Then, using this sorted data, our own personal story is written by the ego.

The ego isn't necessarily a bad thing! It allows us to be functioning individuals and to navigate our experience. But if this is how we understand reality, then the process leaves a lot of room for the ego to fuck around and make it harder for us to see the bigger picture. The ego can blind us to the real story because it's busy narrating its own, where it's the leading character. The ego pushes us further away from reality by doing this, but it just can't help itself. It wants to play the hero role! This enthusiasm makes it easy for the ego to buy into societal script. It reads its lines, believes them, and says, "This is real."

KICK! PUNCH! KARATE CHOP! *CHALLENGE THE SCRIPT.* BE A REBEL.

Unapologetic Awesomeness

Distancing yourself from the Bullshit of the social script is an act of rebellion. By looking at yourself and the world around you with less mist in your eyes, you get closer to reality. This allows you to move forward, not by default but with intention, and opens the doors to becoming unapologetically awesome. I'm not going to candy-coat it; this unapologetically awesome rebellion can be hard at times. Just because you step out of the socially conditioned script doesn't mean other people will stop applying its roles to you. Then again, when your nature is to be majestic as fuck and it doesn't fit the role you're "supposed to" play, what are you supposed to do?

That damned duality can, once again, stick you between a rock and a hard place. It can be difficult to step into your Badass Self, and it can be scary to stand out. Trying to force yourself into a mold that you don't fit can be even more painful, but a lot of us still end up doing that awkward dance. Repeatedly. Just rubbin' all over that mold, trying to shrink and reshape ourselves, and swearing under our breath. Over and over, we hope that finally, just maybe, this time, it'll work. But, uh, isn't that a common definition of insanity? Repeating something over and over and expecting a different result? You bet it is! This duality can drive you up the wall.

There was a time when I desperately, more than anything, wanted to be a dentist. I find it hard to believe now, but it's true! Let me explain.

When I was seven, I cut off my long locks and started spiking my hair. I traded in my dresses for clothes from the boys' section (and immediately got yelled at for being in the girls' washroom). Later, I collected typewriters and, since I had wicked insomnia, would stay up into the wee hours of the morning writing poetry. I wrestled for five years, until all the girls quit when I was thirteen, and eventually, I got bullied by the boys so much that I never left the changing room at practice. I also went for a year without eating with forks out of boredom. When I was asked why this was, I started telling people that forks were a government conspiracy and that the prongs released gases into you that made you want to pay your taxes. I was a "weird" kid.

I was a smart, hypercreative, emotionally unstable kid with no filter and an absent support system. It certainly wasn't the worst hand to be dealt, but I didn't know how to play those cards. I spent a lot of time feeling outside everything. It felt like my strangeness meant swimming upstream 24/7, and I got tired. Eventually, all I wanted was to fit in. I dreamt of having a posh loft apartment; trendy, expensive brand-name sweaters; and white pants that magically always stayed clean. I wanted to be stuck in rush hour so I could bitch about it with my coworkers around the water cooler. I wanted money to buy the things that would make me worthy of acceptance and a title to buy the respect of society.

"Hello! I'm your dentist, Dr. Istace, but you can call me Lindsay."

My attempts to become that person were rough. I did not fit that mold, and it took a toll on me. After a kleptomaniac phase, struggles with substance abuse, battles with mania, depression, and self-harm, I finally hit rock bottom. Getting there was a shitty and wildly educational experience. I definitely had some fun, and I wouldn't trade that time for the world, but I never want to do that again!

One day, after having slept on the street the night before, I found myself in an unfamiliar city with eighteen cents, a green tambourine, a ball, and no way to contact anyone. So I started street performing.

That moment became an important turning point in my life. Long story short: it sent me on a journey that led me back to my authentic self, to my passions, and to people who accepted me. Over time, it brought me to performing professionally, which then gave me opportunities to train and perform all over the world. Eventually, that led me to yoga, and here we are now.

My authentic self had always been creative, playful, strange, and vibrant. When I didn't know how to unapologetically express that, being myself was exhausting and painful as fuck. I had been bullied, rejected, and laughed at. I didn't have a healthy way to deal with that, so I became angry and desperate for relief.

My dream hadn't ever really been to become a dentist. My real dream had simply been to be able to exist comfortably, without the exhaustion and hurt that came from feeling as though I didn't belong. I wanted to play the role of a dentist because it fit into the social script, so I thought it would make my dreams come true. I tried to manipulate and cut out the parts of me that were unsuitable for the role, and it was even harder than being a weirdo. Perhaps dentistry lines up with someone else's authentic self, but that path would have broken me. It took a lot of time and effort, but eventually, I learned to love my strangeness. I discovered that the things about me that had made fitting into the script so hard were actually my biggest assets. I learned to use them to create, connect, and inspire. I wrote my own role, not because of how I thought it would agree with the preexisting script, but because it was the one I was truly made to fill.

Growing into my unapologetically awesome self has been a journey. It has had its own struggles, and sometimes it still does! But I wouldn't have it any other way.

So how exactly does one *be* unapologetically awesome?

AUTHENTICITY + COURAGE = UNAPOLOGETICALLY AWESOME

First, to be authentic, you need to know who you are. So who *are* you?

Authenticity

"To know thyself is the beginning of wisdom." Although it's hard to definitively pin down where it originated, this famous quote is attributed to ancient philosophers. Sound easy, right? It's not. "Who am I?" is a question that has stumped people for a freakin' long time. Some of the most brilliant minds throughout history have gone to the edge of their wits trying to find an answer, only to bring back theoretical clues. So if you think I'm about to hand over the answer on a silver platter, you're going to be sorely disappointed, because those people are a hell of a lot smarter than me!

Still, even if it only brings hypotheses, searching for our own answers is important. There are many things that end up obscuring our real and most Badass Selves, covering them in layers. We have to dig through these layers to get closer to who we truly are.

The Five Koshas

If you invited yogic philosophy over for a potluck, it would bring gluten-free crackers and a forty-layer vegan dip. Every layer of that dip would have its own novel's worth of depth, each with unique layers of spices and textures. Seriously, yogic philosophy *loves* layers! We've already discussed the mind, the intellect, and the ego. These layers allow us to perceive reality and create our personal experiences, but that's where they stop. They don't make us who we are.

We're made of different layers, also referred to *koshas*. Again, the exact terms and number of layers differ between different schools of thought, but the concept is the same: we're like onions. The various yogic systems usually say we have five or seven layers, although the five-layer system seems to be all the rage. This system says that we are not our skin or cells. We are not our brains or our thoughts. Although those are part of us, who we truly are is underneath all those things. These onions have sweet nougat-y centers!

OUR LAYERS LOOK LIKE THIS

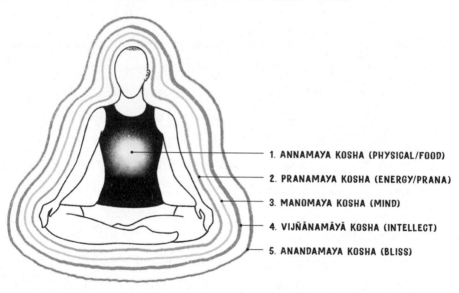

1. ANNAMAYA KOSHA (PHYSICAL/FOOD)
2. PRANAMAYA KOSHA (ENERGY/PRANA)
3. MANOMAYA KOSHA (MIND)
4. VIJÑĀNAMĀYĀ KOSHA (INTELLECT)
5. ANANDAMAYA KOSHA (BLISS)

The first three layers are easy for us to identify, but the ego makes it difficult to dig further. Just like the ego can push reality further away from us when we're perceiving the world, it can push us further away from our true natures as well. It does this the exact same way, by constantly relating itself to the world and narrating the story so it gets to play the hero. The ego builds a false identity by clinging to things like experiences, traits, and labels. By doing so, it attaches us to the outer world and prevents us from getting deeper into that sweet nougat-y center of the real self.

Yogic philosophy would say that none of the identifiers that the ego clings to are real. You can really experience them, but who you are is not composed of them. They would say that *Game of Thrones* is just a TV show. Your favorite sports teams are just people attempting to complete certain activities that someone arbitrarily decided have value. Jobs and passions are just the ways in which you choose to spend your time. Your travel experiences are just you existing in a different geographic location. None of these things really matter, because they are all just part of the illusion. They are not permanent, and they contain no real truth.

At first glance, this seems pretty cold, but it can also be super fucking liberating! It keeps us from obsessing over the unimportant details and opens our eyes to grander things. Imagine straining your eyes and using a magnifying glass to look at a painting. You have no idea what you're look-ing at, and you keep getting closer and closer, trying to see it more clearly. Eventually, you back the fuck up and look again. It's a famous painting, *The Creation of Adam* by Michelangelo. God is reaching out, his fingers nearly meeting Adam's, illustrating the biblical story of man's creation. It's a breathtaking, beautiful, iconic work of art! But you almost missed seeing it because you were zoomed in so close, obsessed with trying to identify one tiny detail. Was it a sand dune or a fortune cookie? No. It was Adam's ball sack.

Go ahead. Geek out over *Game of Thrones*, and get into the game when your favorite sports team plays. Dive into your passions, and remember where you've been. Those things are great! Just be aware that these things can be a trap. If you get wrapped up in the small stuff, you might miss the bigger picture, and you'll catch yourself staring at Adam's ball sack.

It's all right to identify with your passions, relationships, experiences, or what have you. Having a sense of identity is a good thing! However, when it hinges on material world stuff, that sense of identity is fragile. What happens when you finish *Game of Thrones*? When the Cubs lose in the playoffs? When relationships take on new forms or memories fade? Material world things are subject to change at a moment's notice. But dig a little bit deeper, and you find the qualities that compose your authentically Badass Self. That shit is forever!

We can get a better grasp on those qualities by working backward and peeling back the more material labels. For example: I, Lindsay Istace, founded this thing called Rage Yoga. I perform circus arts and dream of opening a circus/yoga center. I want to travel the world to train and learn from kick-ass teachers. I spend a lot of my time making elaborate costumes, training weird circus shit, and doing my personal yoga practices. I am passionate about teaching, watching my students grow, and creating art. None of these things actually define who I am. But when you peel back the layers, you see seeds of truth in there.

There are common threads in my identifiers. Founding Rage Yoga, wanting to open a facility where people can learn, and the joy I get from watching my students grow all point toward me being a teacher. Under that is a seed of nurturing and love. I clearly have a high interest in both arts and circus arts. Performing, teaching, learning, producing...there are many artistic indicators here. Under that is a seed of creativity and playfulness. The love of travel, training, learning, and practicing all show a sense of adventure. That's a seed of curiosity.

So then I, as an animated bag of cells that calls itself a human, am loving, creative, playful, and curious. Sure, the things I spend my time doing will nurture these qualities, but these qualities are what lead me to those other things, not the other way around. They are authentically built into my being, and they say a lot more about who I am than what I do for a living or what I dream about. Those other things matter, but they're more like the leaves that grow when the seeds are cared for.

YOUR SEEDS

What are the things in life that matter to you most? What are the things in your life that you truly identify with? Take that list, and boil it down to its most basic qualities. Rather than the labels or specifics of those things, what are the feelings and motivations behind them? Can you spot any recurring patterns?

Taking a look at ourselves through this lens is a great way to begin operating from a place of authenticity. Not only does it shed a bit of light on the timeless "who am I?" conundrum, but it can remind us to look for the truth and see what is beyond labels and scripts. Doing so will help us be authentic in ourselves, keeping us on the path of unapologetic awesomeness. It reminds us to live intentionally instead of defaulting to autopilot.

Living Intentionally vs. on Autopilot

Everyone has an autopilot setting. It happens when we think, speak, act, or listen without intention. It happens when we think without discerning or speak without minding our words. You can see it when people react without considering their actions or when they listen while only considering their next actions. It's about as authentic as the Mexican cuisine at Taco Bell. Still, Taco Bell is delicious, and this autopilot setting isn't useless!

Operating from an actively observant and discerning place 24/7 isn't possible. Maintaining the high level of focus and presence needed to be fully in the moment is a lot of work, and our attention spans are only so long. Rather than struggling and risking burnout to stay in this intentional state, sometimes you just need to let yourself cruise on autopilot.

Metaphorically speaking, authentic people drive without cruise control as often as they have the energy to. By doing this, they can begin to drive for longer periods of time. They also find that their autopilot setting starts to learn. Rather than just zooming along, crushing mailboxes and frightening children, it gets smarter. Nonmetaphorically speaking, it means that your autopilot mode can be trained so your default self is consistently more badass. This is made possible by working with your authentic mode.

Your authentic mode is very different from your autopilot mode. Living intentionally in your authentic mode is a rebellious act in itself because it distances you from your social conditioning and past behaviors. The more you do this, the easier it will become to spot the weaknesses and holes in your autopilot self. You'll become increasingly aware of your own biases, repeating patterns, and hidden motivations. It's not always easy to look at these things directly, but nothing worth doing is easy! It's just as important to become aware of these imperfect qualities as it is to get to know the seeds of your Badass Self. After all, these imperfect qualities are seeds too.

BADASS HOMEWORK: UNAPOLOGETICALLY AWESOME REALITY CHECK

Note: Use a journal to get the most out of these assignments. It will help you keep track of your thoughts and experiences. If you're not the journal-keeping type, then try reframing it as though you're taking lab notes. Observe yourself with scientific curiosity, and track as much data as you can.

Assignment 1: Check In with Yourself

For the next three days, pay extra attention to your thoughts and actions, observing both your authentic and autopilot modes. How much time do you spend in your authentic mode compared to autopilot? How long do you stay in your authentic mode before you slip back into autopilot?

Our autopilots can teach us a lot about ourselves. While you're tackling this assignment, make sure to reflect on what happened while you were in this mode. What were your thoughts and actions like? Did you find yourself thinking or reacting in ways that you wouldn't choose if you were actively present? This can happen for many different reasons! Past experiences and traumas often influence our responses. Current stressors from one corner of life can spill over into others too. Whatever the cause, these things can make us react strangely or with disproportionate intensity, even if we're not aware of them. So check in!

Do your autopilot behaviors line up with the seed qualities of your Badass Self? If not, what kind of intentional shifts can you make to train your autopilot setting to be more badass?

Note: There are no definitive answers—you're a human, not a sudoku puzzle! That also means the answers you find will change over time, and they won't always be fun. Understanding your inner workings means you're going to kick up some dirt, and that's just part of the process of becoming Zen as fuck. Don't be an asshole to yourself! You're crushing it. Keep it up, you majestic badass!

Assignment 2: Check In with Your World

For the next three days, pay extra attention to what is happening around you in your day-to-day life. Where and how are you spending your time? Who are you spending it with, and what do you do? How do you feel throughout when you do these things? Once you've identified how you spend your time, who you spend it with, and where, ask yourself *why*. Why do you spend your time this way?

You will find that some of these answers are pretty mundane, and that's a-okay. The things that matter to us will always come with their own responsibilities and commitments. To keep those things in our lives, we'll have to take on those responsibilities and commitments. So sometimes we have to do boring shit for the sake of love! But sometimes we take shit on for no good reason. So check in!

Do you spend your time in ways that line up with the seed qualities of your Badass Self? If not, what kind of intentional shifts can you make to reinforce your world and make it more badass?

Imagine you have a garden bed, and in the soil, there is a wide variety of seeds. There is a seed for everything: love, spite, curiosity, anxiety, optimism, sadism, etc. Every time you take an action in life, you water the corresponding seeds. Help a blind stranger cross the street? You probably watered patience, love, and compassion. Kick a dog? You probably just watered ignorance, sadism, and fear. Depending on the hand you were dealt in life and where your autopilot has taken you so far, your garden is bound to have already taken a certain form. Traits you don't want may be taking over, and the ones you do want may be begging for water.

To maintain a healthy garden and keep it in a state that you *actually* want, you need to pay attention to it. You need to know, or at least have a *general idea,* which seeds are planted where and when they need water. You need to care for the plants that grow from the seeds you've watered and pull the weeds you don't want as they pop up. Weeds will pop up! Ignoring them doesn't make them go away; it just lets them grow and choke out the things you want. That's how you get a real shitty garden.

I suck at actual gardening, by the way. A green thumb is not one of my natural strengths. I kill everything! I'm so good at killing plants that friends of mine once gave me rocks painted like cacti as a birthday gift. I'm very aware of how shit I am at gardening, but I'm comfortable with that. No one is perfect. Anyone who tries to convince you otherwise is trying to sell you something or is just really fucking high.

Authentic Imperfection

The ego has a hard time admitting that it's not perfect because it easily (and often) gets wrapped up in pride. After all, it's the hero of the story, dammit! It has rigid expectations about what this hero role looks like, including being good at everything and being right all the time. Because of this, it is *very* sensitive about its imperfections, and it can get irrational when its perfect hero paradigm is challenged. It can be like a toddler screaming "I can't heeeeee-aaaaar yooooooou" after they've been told they can't have another juice box.

Acknowledging our imperfections defuses the awkwardness around them and creates the space to improve. Authentic people own their imperfections instead of becoming owned by them. They work on the parts they want to improve and learn to accept the rest (I don't give a shit about gardening, and I'm not sorry about it). They get good at stuff like admitting weaknesses, owning up to mistakes, and understanding their story as a single thread in a much larger tapestry. When we do these things, we remind the ego that *we* are in control, not the other way around. And no, ego, you can't have another juice box. Keeping the ego in check makes many aspects of life easier to navigate, including conflict.

Someone who is secure in their authenticity is able to be imperfect and willing to be wrong. This means they don't need to win an argument to validate themselves! They know other people's views don't negate their own, so they can comfortably listen to contrasting values and opinions. In fact, they are so secure in themselves that they can see value in opposing views, even if they don't agree with them as a whole. They don't try to force the world into the shape of their ego because they understand that their individual reality is not universally true or perfect. This raw authenticity is potent stuff, and it is the secret sauce that can make conflict productive.

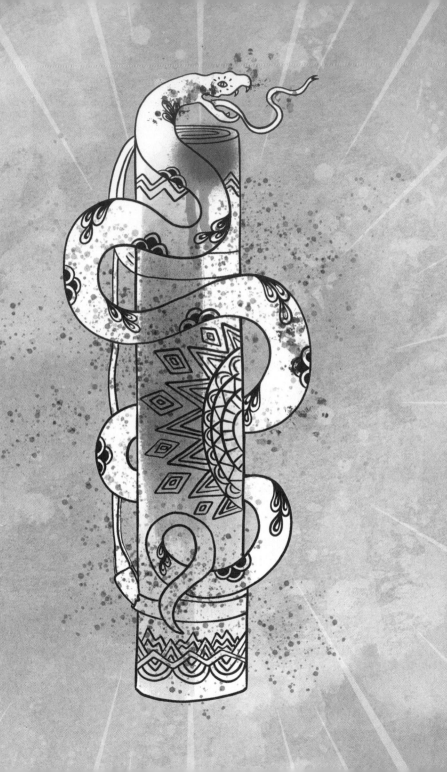

5

LIVE
FEARLESSLY

"Be confused, it's where you begin to learn new things.
Be broken, it's where you begin to heal. Be frustrated,
it's where you start to make more authentic decisions.
Be sad, because if we are brave enough, we can hear
our heart's wisdom though it. Be whatever you are
right now. No more hiding. You are worthy, always."
—S. C. LOURIE

Quick recap: authenticity + courage = unapologetically awesome.

We've talked authenticity. Now let's talk courage.

The first step to being courageous is being vulnerable. Seems coun-
terintuitive, right? We've been given some really backward messages about
what vulnerability means. It's often thought of like being a turtle on its

back, soft belly up in the air, helpless and exposed to danger. The ego doesn't like this look because a hero is supposed to be able to defend themselves; that's just what heroes do! We want to be and see courageous and confident badasses, but we rarely get to see what that functionally looks like. The truth is that the characteristics we admire in these badasses aren't innate givens. They're results of well-tended seeds of vulnerability.

Vulnerability Is Hard-Core

Vulnerability is fucking hard-core! Every time you step outside your comfort zone, you make yourself vulnerable because you're exposed to the possibilities of failure, rejection, and criticism. Sometimes you're exposed to these possibilities even when you're *inside* your comfort zone. You won't get hit every time you make yourself vulnerable, but *it will happen*, and sometimes it's going to hurt like hell.

When we experience this kind of hurt, the ego does everything it can to minimize the pain and keep us from similar ouchy-ness in the future. No matter how true it might be, it begins by writing a story to explain how the hero was wrongly victimized. Next, it programs new autopilot responses. These responses are rarely helpful, and they tend to push us further away from our authentic mode of being. Even if it means developing new habits or traits that are harmful to us in other ways, the ego wants to shower us in armor and protect us at all costs. Rather than risk vulnerability or face hurt in a constructive way, the ego wants to hide from it.

The mark of real badasses is that when the shit hits the fan, they stay vulnerable instead of allowing themselves to be crushed under a mountain of armor. They grow from the experience, taking away lessons from the highs and the lows, so they can improve next time. They don't intentionally seek out potentially painful situations, but they certainly don't shy away from them. Real badasses are strong enough to allow themselves to hurt. Their armor is their vulnerability, and it will protect them more than any defenses that the ego could provide. Vulnerability isn't weakness; it's fucking courageous. Vulnerability is the absence of fear.

Fear

So what is fear then? It's a survival instinct. It's one of the most basic emotions we have, which means there are a lot of seeds o' fear planted in our gardens. It's important to keep an eye out for them and tend to them as they pop up, and they will pop up! It's inevitable. Most often, they show up as feelings of anxiety, humiliation, rejection, worthlessness, and insecurity.

An unapologetic badass doesn't shy away from fear. They look at it head-on, examining it to see what its true shape is, because just like us, fear has layers. You might say that you're afraid of public speaking, but that's just the surface layer. If you peel that back, you'll see that you're actually afraid of something else. It's not public speaking; it's the fact that it opens you up to humiliation and criticism if it doesn't go the way you want.

 BADASS HOMEWORK: DISMANTLE YOUR FEAR

We all have an emotional reality and a logical one. They both exist at the same time and in the same brain, but they often only have a tiny corner of overlap. Taking time to analyze your fears will help you make sense of them and give you insights on how to move past them. People are afraid of all sorts of things, and we usually spend more energy avoiding our fears than we would if we actually faced them. So first you gotta ask yourself, "What am I afraid of?"

Writing about it is helpful, and "free writing" is your best friend! Type in an empty Word document or grab a piece of paper, and let your unfiltered thoughts pour out. Don't let yourself get hung up on silly things like spelling or sentence structure. Don't worry if it makes sense. Just. Write. Let your inner dialogue flow continuously, and you will find some li'l truth nuggets amid the word vomit. Once you've identified some of your fears, you may want to go one step further and peel back that surface layer. What is your fear really about? Do you have an idea of where it comes from?

Now let's get a little sci-fi up in here... Your clone is sitting next to you. Yes, it's only human nature to challenge your clone to a death match, but you must fight this impulse. Your clone is struggling with the same fears you have and is worried about the same shit that's on your mind. They need your support and are asking for advice. What kind of guidance do you give them, and how do you talk to them?

Sitting around and having full-blown back-and-forth conversations with yourself can feel a little weird at first, but it gets results! Most people find it easy to empathize and lift up others. Many do so instinctually. However, we often have a hard time extending these things to ourselves, so we become our own bullies instead. When we take a step back to support our clones, we're more likely to treat ourselves the same way we would treat others. It can also defuse the emotional chaos that's tied to our fears, so we can see through it more clearly.

You can feel fear in your body when your heart rate increases. You lose your breath, and maybe your palms get sweaty or you feel nauseous. It feels super fucking real, yet fear is an intangible thing! Although we can feel its effects, it can't physically touch us. Sometimes our fears have very real origin stories. Other times they are just the ego manically writing irrational stories in an effort to stay in control so it can have that "hero" narrative that it's so fucking horny for. Either way, it's not a literal monster, crouching in the shadows, waiting to attack us with its razor talons as soon as we make ourselves vulnerable.

The power that fear has over us is amplified by how badly we want to avoid it. Don't look at it. Don't think about. Do *not* talk about it. Hiding in denial can offer some shred of temporary comfort, but it screws us in the long run. That's how fear starts looking like actual monsters crouching in the corners of our eyes. Big or small, the things that scare us lose a lot of their power once we acknowledge them. For example, once Harry Potter started referring to He Who Shall Not Be Named by his real name, Lord Voldemort (or Tom Marvolo Riddle), that son of a bitch lost some of the power he had gained by causing fear.

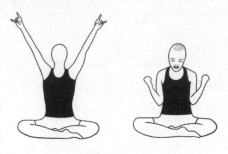

VICTORY BREATHS

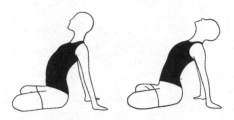

SEATED CHEST OPENER

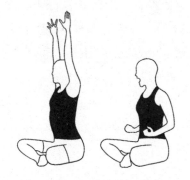

SEATED FISTS OF FIRE

Get started by sitting down on your mat and doing five to ten Victory Breaths. Let your chest really expand on your inhales and lift your gaze like a mother fuckin' rock star. On your exhales think about pulling all of that badass confidence in, compacting and absorbing it into you. Next, find some stillness in a Seated Chest Opener for five breaths. Feel your chest lifting and expanding on every inhale, basking in this posture. If it feels right, smile! Move on to five to ten Seated Fists of Fire. Inhale Good Shit. Exhale Bullshit. Inhale confidence and exhale self doubt.

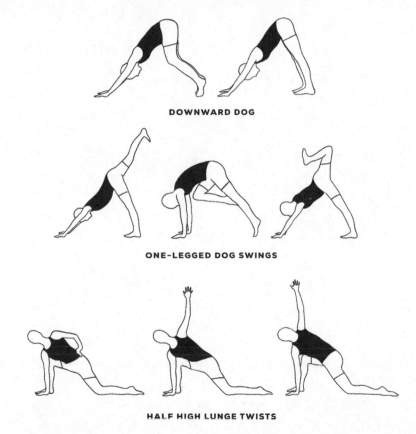

DOWNWARD DOG

ONE-LEGGED DOG SWINGS

HALF HIGH LUNGE TWISTS

Come onto all fours, curl your toes under and toward the front of your mat, then lift up into Downward Dog. Stay here for three breaths, mentally scanning your body and thanking it for its strength. Lift one leg and begin three to five One-Legged Dog Swings, feeling the ease of your inhales and the power of your exhales. Plant the foot of your swinging leg up by your hands and come into Half High Lunge. Stay here for three breaths and then begin Half High Lunge Twists. Twist one direction for three breaths, then twist the other direction for another three.

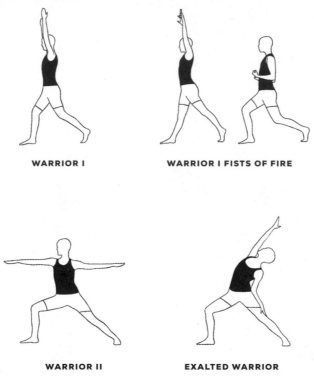

WARRIOR I

WARRIOR I FISTS OF FIRE

WARRIOR II

EXALTED WARRIOR

Curl your back toes under and toward the front of your mat and then, moving boldly with your breath, rise into Warrior I. Begin three to five Warrior I Fists of Fire, courageously lifting with your inhales and powerfully contracting as you lower with your exhales. Bring your hands up overhead, then exhale as you come into Warrior II like the super suave badass that you are. Stay strong here, keeping your spine tall and gaze slightly lifted, for three to five breaths. If you like, you can add some extra attitude by tossing up some fist unicorns. Next, exhale as you engage your core and lean back in Exalted Warrior. Take three to five deep breaths in this pose, embodying triumph like a freakin' champion!

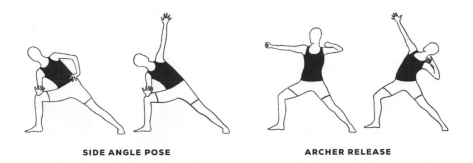

SIDE ANGLE POSE　　　　　　　**ARCHER RELEASE**

Bring your torso back up and over to get into Side Angle Pose. Hold this pose for three to five breaths, lifting confidently through your core and perhaps sending your gaze up to the sky. Lifting up and over once again, lean back and begin Archer Release. Inhale the Good Shit with every prep, bringing in more of whatever it is that you need to conquer your fear. Exhale the Bullshit with every release, letting go of any thoughts or beliefs that are getting in your way. If it feels good, then get loud with it! Let it be cathartic as fuck and keep it up for five breaths.

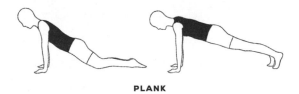

PLANK

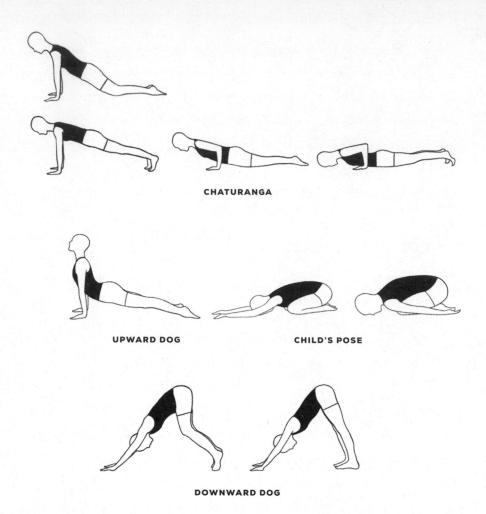

CHATURANGA

UPWARD DOG   **CHILD'S POSE**

DOWNWARD DOG

Let your arms windmill forward and down to the mat, bringing your hands out to the sides of your feet. Power up your core as you step the front foot back by the other to come into Plank Pose. Keep this powerful engagement through your body as you move through Chaturanga. Once you've arrived on the mat, rest your forehead and take a breath to pause and steep in the victories of what you've accomplished. These accomplishments could be things you've done off the mat, out in the world, or the fact that you've made it this far through this sequence. When you're ready, push through your hands and lift through your core as you come into Upward Dog, holding the pose for three breaths. Then, on your exhale, bring your badass booty back to your heels and move into Child's Pose. Breathe, badass, breathe. When you wanna, bring yourself into Downward Dog.

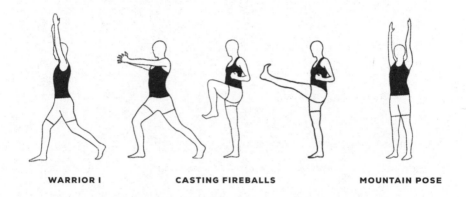

WARRIOR I   **CASTING FIREBALLS**   **MOUNTAIN POSE**

Lift one leg up high, charging it with the energy of your inhale, then, following the rhythm of your exhale, carry that energy forward to plant your foot by your hands. Rise up with your breath into Warrior I. Steady yourself here, grounding into your feet and your Badass Self. Begin Casting Fireballs for a total of five... or more if you're feeling it! You're the boss. On your last fireball, step your lifted foot down to come into a strong Mountain Pose. Inhale your hands up high overhead, then bring them down to the center of your chest. Give yourself a "fuck yeah!" You deserve it.

By looking at our fears, we can start to learn about them. We can learn about where they come from and how to ease them. In this process, we end up dismantling them and decreasing their power over us. Dismantling them also gives us an incredible opportunity to harvest some power of our own. None of this applies solely to fear. This is all true of every ouchy emotion we are capable of feeling!

Our uncomfortable emotions can act as bumpers that alert us when we're off course. They can remind us that we're not properly caring for our health or our happiness, or that we're disconnected from our Badass Selves. Being honest about our emotions makes it possible for us to receive these internal guiding memos. This vulnerability also allows us to heal and grow from less-than-awesome experiences.

Painful emotions are like a never-ending dance, and real badasses do their best to study the steps. Instead of getting knocked around the dance floor, they learn how to move gracefully through it. It's necessary if you want to lead a Zen as fuck life! Even then, not even the most baddest of asses is completely immune. But when they miss their steps and get knocked around, they stay vulnerable. This means they get a huge resistance boost against things like fear. It also keeps their egos in check.

The ego often uses our painful emotions to control us. Again, it's a super annoying and misguided attempt to protect us. By working through the ego's Bullshit, we have a chance to take back the wheel and choose our own direction. Buckled into the back seat, the ego will still make some snide remarks, but it doesn't get to choose the destination.

So what now, badass?

Fear be damned, where do you wanna go?

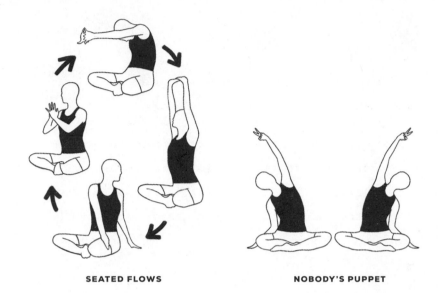

SEATED FLOWS   **NOBODY'S PUPPET**

Get yourself into a comfortable seated position and begin Seated Flows. Supercharge your inhales to find some extra expansion and lift through your chest. Once you've repeated this flow three to five times, ground your Badass Self in stillness for a couple breaths. Moving into Nobody's Puppet, feel your breath coming into your side body as you reach up and over. Moving with your breath, picture cutting those puppet strings as you move from side to side, freeing yourself of patterns and expectations that dull your unapologetically awesome self. Don't apologize, just cut those fucking strings five times.

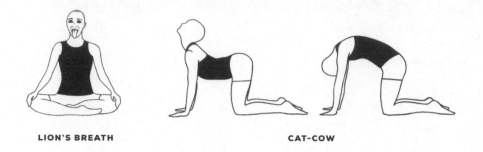

LION'S BREATH

CAT-COW

Begin Lion's breath. Stick your tongue aaaaaallll the way out and open your eyes as wide as possible, letting your exhales come out through your mouth. Let those exhales be LOUD! Does it look silly? Probably. Do you give a shit? Hell no! Repeat this breath five times. Bring yourself up onto all fours and follow your breath as you move through Cat-Cow five to seven times.

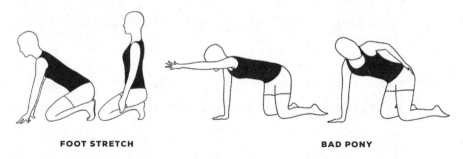

FOOT STRETCH

BAD PONY

Curl your toes under and toward the top of your mat. Bring your hips back, sitting on your heels as you come into a Foot Stretch. Letting your shoulders relax and keeping your spine long, stay here for five breaths. Back on all fours, begin being one super Bad Pony! Feel the lift and expansion through your body on every inhale. Feel the engagement of your muscles on every exhale, as you bend to the side and give dat booty a tap of unapologetic appreciation. Repeat five times on both sides.

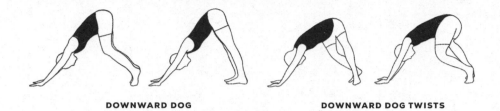

DOWNWARD DOG　　　　　　　　**DOWNWARD DOG TWISTS**

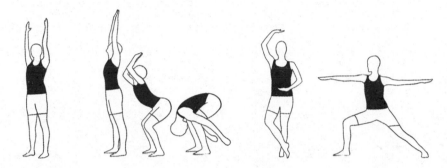

MOUNTAIN POSE　　**LET THAT SHIT GO BREATH**　　**BOB'S COSMIC DANCER**　　**WARRIOR II**

Curl your toes under and lift your hips up into Downward Dog. Stay here for three breaths. Begin to move freely, following your breath, as you begin Downward Dog Twists. Twist in this position as long as it feels good! You make the rules, badass. Once you're satisfied, step or hop your feet up to your hands. In this position, all curled up and folded, find your center of gravity. Keep this center in mind as you slowly rise to a standing position, rolling your body up and open, coming into Mountain Pose. Anchor into yourself, grounding through your feet, lengthening your spine, and relaxing your shoulders. Let this grounded feeling soak in, and stay here as long as you need. Then start Let That Shit Go Breath. Bring your hands up overhead, expanding and building yourself tall with your inhale. On your exhale...let that shit go unapologetically! Let gravity do its thing as you flop forward and bring your hands to the mat. Repeat three to five times. Back in a standing position, shift your weight into one foot, lifting the other, and come into Bob's Cosmic Dancer. Lengthen your spine, standing tall like the badass that you are, and ground down through your supporting foot. Feeling fancy? Try experimenting with your arm positions or testing out some mudras. Revel in this posture for five breaths. Next, step your lifted foot back and move into Warrior II. Keep your posture tall and gaze over your front middle finger...and feel free to turn that finger up for extra sass! Lift your chin slightly and hold here for three breaths.

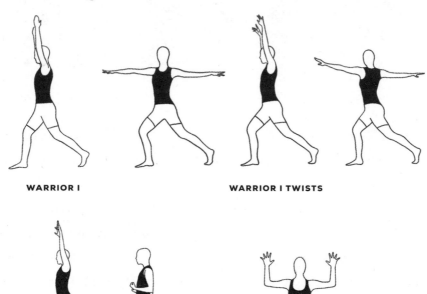

WARRIOR I   **WARRIOR I TWISTS**

WARRIOR I FISTS OF FIRE   **GODDESS POSE**

Rage Yoga

Rotating from the hip, turn your back leg so your toes point to the front of your mat. Inhale and bring your hands over head, coming into Warrior I. Steady yourself here, then begin Warrior I Twists. As you twist each way, imagine sending energy out through your arms to open them wide and create extra space for your chest to expand. Twist each way three times, then bring yourself back to your neutral starting position. Commence Warrior I Fists of Fire! Let your inhales lift you as you straighten your legs. Bend your legs as you pull your arms down and in on your exhales. Keep your chin lifted and make some noise! Don't hold anything back. Repeat this breath three to five times, you majestic badass. Next, step your back foot a little closer to the back of your mat. Come up onto the balls of your feet and turn your body to the open side of your mat. Exhale as you bend your knees and come into Goddess Pose. Be your Badass Self here for three breaths.

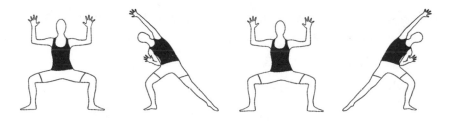

GODDESS REACHES

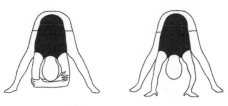

WIDE-LEGGED FORWARD FOLD

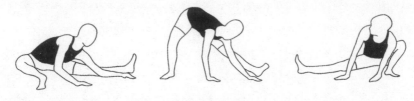

NINJA LUNGES

Begin Goddess Reaches, shifting from one foot to the other and lengthening your side body. Reach to each side five to seven times, keeping your gaze lifted and staying steady in your breath. Return to your neutral starting position, then let your upper body melt down. Bring your hands to the mat and come into Wide-Legged Forward Fold. Don't rush this pose. You don't owe this time to anyone but yourself. Let your upper body be heavy, take your arms to wherever feels natural, and just let yourself marinate in this awesome sauce. At your leisure, leave your feet in place as you lower your hips to begin Ninja Lunges. Follow your instincts and play around, moving side to side through these lunges for five to seven breaths.

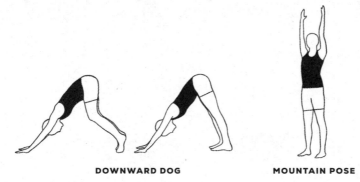

DOWNWARD DOG   **MOUNTAIN POSE**

Walk your hands to the front of your mat and shift your feet to come into Downward Dog. Feel the lift as your lungs expand with your inhales and focus on your strength radiating from your core and through your limbs on your exhales. Hold here for three breaths. Next, step, or jump, or hop your feet up to your hands. Stack yourself over your center of gravity and then slowly roll up with your breath into a Mountain Pose. Lift your hands overhead with your inhale, then bring them down to the center of your chest with your exhale. Give yourself an authoritative and unapologetic "fuck yeah!"

Creating Your Badass Reality

I don't know about you, but I'm super sick of hearing people talk about the *magic* of "manifesting your destiny." The general idea is awesome, but it often gets fluffed up and watered down. As a result, there are a lot of people waiting around, reeking of patchouli, expecting the universe to magically hand over the things they want. Although I personally love the smell of patchouli, I do not buy into the idea that you can magically just *think* things into existence. Things don't come to you simply by daydreaming about them or because it's "destined." The universe doesn't owe you shit. Still, regardless of your opinions on astrology and patchouli, you can create the life and experiences you want. But you'll need a plan.

Buckle up, badass! We're about to break it down.

Are you ready?

Seven Steps to Creating Your Badass Reality

1. Know what you want.
2. Get stoked.
3. Do the work and parkour that shit.
4. Learn, trust, and look foolish.
5. Pay attention!
6. Don't be a dick.
7. Stay out of your own way.

Know What You Want

Again, you can't simply think the things you want into reality! However, you do need to know what you want, so thinking about those things is hugely important. Put real thought and time into this, and consider your goals carefully before locking them in. Are they really what you want? Are they truly *your* goals, or are you designing your reality around what other people want for you or around what you're *supposed* to want? Be honest with yourself so you can avoid spending your precious fucks on something that doesn't actually support your Badass Self.

Doing actual research about your goal is also important. Talk to people, pick up some books, hit up Google, etc. Arm yourself with knowledge, and answer some questions before you get to work. When the thing you want is a reality, will it be one that you actually want, or is it just nice to think about? What are you going to need to learn, and what kind of steps are you going to have to take? What is required to maintain that reality once you get there? Are these things that you're willing to do, or are you going to be miserable the entire time?

You don't need to have *all* the answers before setting out, but you should have at least some idea of what you're getting yourself into! Otherwise, you could end up several hundred dollars poorer, with an enormous collection of materials and tools, only to discover that you fucking hate sewing. Then that pile of stuff might sit around for a painfully long time while you quietly beat yourself up about it every time you see it until finally, years later, you give it away to someone who will actually use it. Not that this suspiciously specific example has ever happened to me...

Once you've locked in that target goal, keep learning about it. Know the thing you want so well that you can smell, hear, and even taste it. Imagine exactly what that outcome looks and feels like. Being able to visualize it clearly is helpful because it teaches your mind that you can have it. You are capable and you're allowed, dammit! It also keeps it in the forefront of your mind, which will help you stay focused and excited about it.

Get Stoked

Some people say that you shouldn't talk about what you're doing until it's done. I say, "Fuck that!" Light that fire, and let it burn bright. Let yourself get excited. Daydream about it. Talk about it. This reaffirms that what you're doing isn't impossible nonsense—it's real.

Talking about it might feel weird or forced at first, and you might worry that people aren't taking you seriously. You might even have a hard time taking yourself seriously at first! However, as long as you're taking steps to get there (even if they're just small steps), you won't just be talking about it with empty words. You'll be sharing your process with other people and giving them the opportunity to see you on your journey. You'll be giving them the chance to support you by believing in you, cheering you on, or simply being there. Your enthusiasm will also lead you to people who are willing to share their own experiences or resources, which can help you chart unfamiliar territory. Whatever it is you've set your sights on, you won't be able to get there alone. In-person and online, there are experts and communities for everything, so get out there and talk about it!

Do the Work and Parkour That Shit

After all that thinking, researching, dreaming, and talking, you have to actually do something about it. If you catch yourself feeling overwhelmed by the big picture, break it down into bite-size pieces. Every journey starts with a single step. Breathe. The more frequently you step outside your comfort zone, the easier it gets and the bigger your comfort zone becomes. Taking any action, even if small, makes fear quieter. Fearless action crushes it.

Speaking of fearlessly crushing it... You've probably seen videos of people doing parkour, courtesy of the internet. If you haven't, get on that! It's a sport where people move through spaces in the most ninja-like way possible. They can be walking through an everyday place like a train station, and they'll do it while running up walls, swinging off signs, and doing backflips off tables. If you do parkour, kudos to you! That shit is awesome. It looks super fun, and if I had better health insurance, I'd definitely try it out myself. Why the hell not? If you're going somewhere anyway, why not have the most fun you can while getting there? Does the distance between point A and B have to be so monotonous? In a similar fashion, since you're already undertaking this journey toward your goals, why not do some mental parkour? There is a lot of hard work ahead. You'll probably run into some obstacles and have to endure some tedious shit, but does it all have to feel like a grind? You're already heading that way so...parkour!

Learn, Trust, and Look Foolish

There's a wise saying that I've seen many times on inspirational posters and home decor from Hallmark. I've heard it from the mouths of celebrity speakers, teachers, and porn stars in adult films. "To get results you've never had, you have to do something you've never done." They've got a point.

If you're working toward obtaining a life you haven't had before, you're going be doing many new things. Wiring in new habits, learning new skills, and stepping outside your comfort zone are all parts of the learning process! Throughout that process, you're going to fuck up and catch yourself looking like an idiot. That is just how learning works, my friend. My time in the circus world has proven to me, time and time again, that this is so true it's almost comedic.

Have you ever seen a juggling act that is so incredible you forget to breathe? I have several friends who perform at that level, and they are amazing to watch! They look like fucking superheroes when you see them onstage, but the audience never sees the amount of practice it takes to get there. A juggler isn't born a juggler! It. Takes. Work. Yeah, they smile and make it look oh so easy onstage now, but at one point, they looked like complete fools!

At first, a juggler is just a person who wants to learn to juggle. They know what it looks like, but they have zero experience. They spend countless hours, swearing under their breath and chasing balls around a room, concentrating so hard that they look like they may have shit themselves. They get a tiny bit better, and then somehow, they get worse. If you need to get past them, you just wait for them to stop because you don't trust their skills enough to be closer than ten feet. But they keep at it! Eventually, they get good. Then one day, because why not, you lie underneath them on a white carpet and drink red wine from a delicate glass while they juggle over your head.

The jugglers of the world worked through frustration and exhaustion, through looking foolish, and they didn't quit when it was hard. They kept picking up those damn balls and trying again. With or without juggling balls, this is true for anyone who has ever become good at anything. They had to start with zero experience and trust that their skill would improve.

You don't need to be an expert right fucking now. You just need to trust that it'll all come in time because, quite simply, it will! The ego will always be the number one roadblock to learning and growing. It doesn't like the vulnerability involved. Just keep showing up. Do the work, learn fearlessly, and don't be afraid to look authentically foolish.

Pay Attention!

When opportunity knocks, answer the damn door! Don't let it pass by, because opportunity rarely leaves messages. You need to be ready and willing to let it in when it arrives, so be prepared. You wouldn't sit in the basement watching Netflix with noise-canceling headphones on if you were expecting a guest, would you?

True story: I was recently expecting a friend of mine to show up at my place to pick something up. I was waiting by the door and writing. Writing this book, in fact! There was a knock. I opened the door and was suddenly surprised. There was a beautiful shirtless person in my doorway with a boa constrictor wrapped around their shoulders. It was the friend I'd been waiting for, just...well, y'know. She had less clothing and more snakes on than I had expected. Why and how could I possibly have been expecting it? It was still my fabulous friend but, I have to honest, it took me a minute to realize who she was.

Similarly, when opportunity shows up at your door, it might not look exactly like you thought it would. That doesn't mean the universe is cat-fishing you or that it'll show up with a snake. It just means that you need to pay extra attention, or you might not recognize it.

You can often have one plan when life has another. Like sailing on open waters, things can be calm and steady, but you can bet your ass it won't stay that way forever! There will be waves, currents, and weather you can't predict. If you're paying attention and keeping control of your sails, *you will get to where you want to be.* You might just end up arriving a little differently than you had expected. Taking a different course or landing a little off target doesn't mean you've failed. Instead of losing your shit and stubbornly battling forces you can't control, stay flexible in your expectations. You'll find it's easier to stay true to your destination. Plus, you'll get to relax and enjoy the scenery more.

Getting too wrapped up in the *right-fucking-now* while pursuing your goals can make you forget to stop and enjoy yourself. You can also run the risk of becoming so obsessed with your destination that you're oblivious to your own progress. It's like spending a bunch of time and energy to plant and care for a garden but not appreciating it when the seeds begin to sprout. What're you waiting for? A lush garden to just pop up all at once? Is *that* when you're going to feel that your effort has value? Is *that* when you're going to be happy? Nah! Enjoy your garden as it comes to life. Get curious as it grows, love it as it blossoms, and take pride as it produces fruit. Or vegetables. Or flowers, or whatever the hell you planted. I'm not your dad. It's your garden; you should know!

Don't Be a Dick

Don't be a dick!

Seems like it should be easy enough, right? You might be surprised.

Even really good people can turn into real assholes when they get too focused on themselves. The reality is that any form of introspection or work that someone does to build a reality they want means spending a lot of time looking inward. You'll probably find that you think about yourself a lot. If you don't keep an eye on this, you run the risk of becoming a selfish dick.

Being selfish is not always a bad thing. In fact, it can be necessary! Discerning how you spend your time, attention, and energy is healthy. Budgeting these things will conserve your precious fucks so you can spend them wisely on the things and people that really matter to you. You can't expect to be happy or to reach your goals if you have an overspent fuck budget.

Selfishness becomes bad when you get so hyperfocused on yourself and your goals that you start taking other aspects of your life for granted. This happens when the ego crawls out of the back seat, gets ahold of the wheel, and starts driving you into its hero narrative. Your viewpoint gets narrowed down so much that all you can see is yourself and what is immediately in front of you. It can make you forget about the awesome people in your life and the good things that you already have. In this obsessive state, it's easy to become restless and insensitive and to alienate the people you care about. You can spend all the time and energy in the world to create something beautiful, but if you become a dick along the way, you can push away the people you wanted to share it with.

Stay Out of Your Own Way

One of the biggest things that often stands in our way is ourselves. While loudly insisting that we're the heroes of our own stories, the ego can turn us into the baddest of villains. This isn't the good kind of bad, like *"Oh, girl, you are bad!"* This is the full-blown cape-wearing, puppy-dog-stealing, baby-cursing kind of bad.

The ego loves a thick plot and dramatic hero's journey. So especially when things are going well for us, it can be tempted to introduce a villain to come in and complicate things. Why? The short answer is because it can be a real asshole! The long answer is because it believes that heroes have to struggle, because just like in the movies, their stories end once the conflict is resolved. They ride off into the sunset, the credits roll, and then it's over. So the ego must have a villain—or invent one—so the hero can keep on hero-ing. The core belief here is "I struggle, therefore I am." There has to be a conflict to overcome and a struggle in order to prevail... Just look at the codependent relationship between Batman and the Joker! They need each other to reinforce their own identities (and, by extension, probably their self-worth as well).

The mind is simultaneously our greatest ally and our biggest adversary. So it makes sense that we regularly get the opportunity to play both hero and villain in our own personal stories, cycling back and forth and back again. This can result in a cycle of self-sabotage. These cycles can be tricky to spot and even more challenging to break out of. They become subconscious habits, because although it's clearly fucked up, the ego genuinely believes it's keeping us safe. It knows you lived through these trials last time and, my goodness, you looked so heroic overcoming them! So it puts you back there again because it believes that anything, any-fucking-thing, is safer than change. Misery, mediocrity, abuse...you name it!

To overcome self-sabotage, you first need to spot it. Addiction, commitment issues, crippling self-doubt, and procrastination are common forms of self-sabotage, but it's not exactly a one-size-fits-all kind of scenario. These cycles are generally born out of personal traumas and fear, so they can look very different from person to person. Locating them is like finding a weed in your garden. Somehow, a seed found its way into your garden and, in one way or another, was nurtured enough to grow into a full-blown Bullshit plant. No need to panic. Weeds happen! The most important thing is that you tend to your garden and pay attention so you notice if it pops back up. Some weeds are more deep rooted and invasive than others and require more vigilance.* When you do the work to weed out your internal obstacles, the external obstacles become easier to move as well.

These seven steps are not *magic*. It's way the fuck more effort than simply waving a wand or thinking nice thoughts until things show up on a silver platter, but these steps deliver results. They are a solid and very real method to achieving the badass reality you want. They can bring you incredible rewards, inside and out. It isn't always fun or easy, but it does get easier the more you do it!

There is a concept in Buddhism that is often referred to as the "practice of nonpractice." The idea is that when you intentionally shape your thoughts, words, and actions in a certain fashion, you eventually start to do the thing without much intentional work on your part. In other words, you train your autopilot response. At first, it takes some work to curate your thoughts, words, and actions. Once there, even if just for moments at a time, you find that fantastic sweet spot, and it all happens naturally. The more you find that sweet spot, the easier it is to get there and stay there for longer. That little sweet spot is kind of like a clitoris. It's small and can be tricky to find, and some people don't even know what it looks like! Once you locate it, you need to learn how to work it, and that can feel awkward at first. Just like a clitoris, when properly worked, this sweet spot of nonpractice comes with a lot of naturally flowing power and potential that can be overwhelming.

---

* Some things can't be done alone. This is hard stuff, so don't be afraid to ask for help if you need it! If you find the right one, therapists are great at mind gardening.

Don't Get Held Back

Unapologetic badasses tend to stick out. They have an authentic vulnerability and strength to them. They fearlessly create and advocate for the reality they want, and it's fucking cool! But, uh, it's not really a role that the social script has prepared for, and it can rub some people the wrong way. You'll encounter people who find you to be "too much" in one way or another. Maybe they just think you're too intense or find you intimidating. Often when people have a hard time living the life they want, they find it challenging to be around those who are. Some people will find it inspiring, but others will start comparing themselves. Comparing ourselves to others is an ego game that can cause several different reactions. Some people might go into self-deprecation mode, and others might go into attack mode. Whatever reaction they might have to you, don't compromise your awesomeness to make other people comfortable!

It's important to consider the comfort and feelings of the people around us. Without those things, we stop being unapologetic badasses and become self-absorbed assholes. Remember, there is a big difference between being authentically confident and being an obnoxious egomaniac. But consideration for others can go too far and become an unhealthy reflex when we assume complete responsibility for their feelings and reactions. Sometimes you can trigger discomfort in people because of their own baggage, and that's not your fault or your problem. Sometimes people can just flat out not like you, and that's not your fault or your problem either.

If you feel as though you're "too much" and are changing your behavior in response to that, ask yourself if it's genuinely out of consideration or an instinct to please people. People pleasing is a trap. It causes us to amputate the most real and interesting parts of ourselves in exchange for someone else's behaviors, beliefs, or expectations. This usually happens in an attempt to avoid conflict and gain approval, which is understandable. Conflict is stressful, and approval is comforting. Still, people pleasing is pointless. No matter how much of our "muchness" we saw off and no matter how many inoffensive traits we adopt, we will never be liked universally. *Nothing is ever liked universally.*

Have you ever hung out with a group of friends or been to a function where food is ordered for everyone? It's complicated, because beyond just their preferences, you have to plan around everyone's intolerances, allergies, and dietary restrictions. Pizza usually ends up being the safest bet, specifically cheese pizza. I can't tell you how many events I've been to where cheese pizza is the only food that everyone can agree on, but no one is actually happy about it.

Elbert Hubbard once said, "To escape criticism: do nothing, say nothing, be nothing." Although I have no idea what his pizza tastes were like, he would agree that even cheese pizza, the safest and most universal of foods, can't be loved by everyone. There are people out there who truly detest cheese pizza, even though it has done nothing besides simply existing. You don't even have to be doing anything worthwhile; doing anything at all means you're going to face criticism. Why waste your time trying to make yourself palatable enough to avoid criticism?

When you unleash your Badass Self, you're going to make some waves. Friends and family can quickly grow closer or further apart from you. New people in your life will be either quickly repelled or immediately attracted. You're not going to be cheese pizza. You're going to be one of those artisan hipster pizzas, and that's going to get you some polarizing reactions. Those who are into it are *really fucking into it*. Focus on these people, because they clearly have great taste. As for those who don't like what you're serving, let them go! Or at the very least, let their opinions go.

BADASS HOMEWORK: WHO ARE YOUR PEOPLE?

Assignment 1: What's Your Average?

Who are the five people you spend the most time with?

Write their names down, then add answers to the following questions for each person.

What are their most predominant qualities that stand out to you?

Are there things you admire about them?

Are there things about them that make you uncomfortable?

You are the average of these people. Is the average of these people an outcome that supports your Badass Self? Hopefully, the answer is yes! But if you find yourself spending time and energy with people who do not contribute positively to an average that you want to be, you may want to consider making some adjustments. People curate aspects of their lives all the time. They curate the art in their homes, the clothes in their wardrobes, the food in their fridges, and so on. However, we don't always think about the necessity of curating the people in our lives.

Assignment 2: Your Top Five

Who are the five people you are truly closest with? These may not be the people you see all the time, for one reason or another. These are people you deeply respect. They make you feel safe and loved, and their presence in your life means a lot to you. Write their names down.

Second to your own, these are the only people whose opinions matter. Don't waste your time bending over backward and compromising yourself for people who aren't on this list. If other people don't like your particular brand of awesome, that's a them problem.

This can all be a lot of work, but it's amazing how much of that work can be boiled down to just letting go! Letting go of expectations, ego, fear, and Bullshit in general allows us to clear the way and step into our Badass Selves. Our Badass Selves are Zen as fuck! When we're operating from this place, it is so much easier to live fearlessly and to create the realities we want.

This real-life magical place of Badass Self has always been there and will continue to always be there. You didn't just read a book about Rage Yoga that magically fixed you so you can feel awesome. You have *always* been awesome and will continue to *always* be awesome. All your flaws, shortcomings, and struggles do not make you broken or "less than." You are not awesome *in spite* of these things. You're just awesome.

You deserve love, confidence, and happiness. You deserve good things. Damn it, you majestic badass, you are worthy.

YOU DO NOT NEED ANYONE ELSE'S PERMISSION TO FEEL THESE THINGS!

You sure as fuck don't need it, but for whatever it's worth, you absolutely have my permission.

Can I get a "Fuck yeah!"?

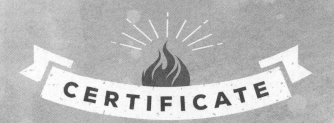

CERTIFICATE

I HEREBY GRANT

_____

_____

YOUR NAME HERE

PERMISSION TO BE

MAJESTIC AS FUCK

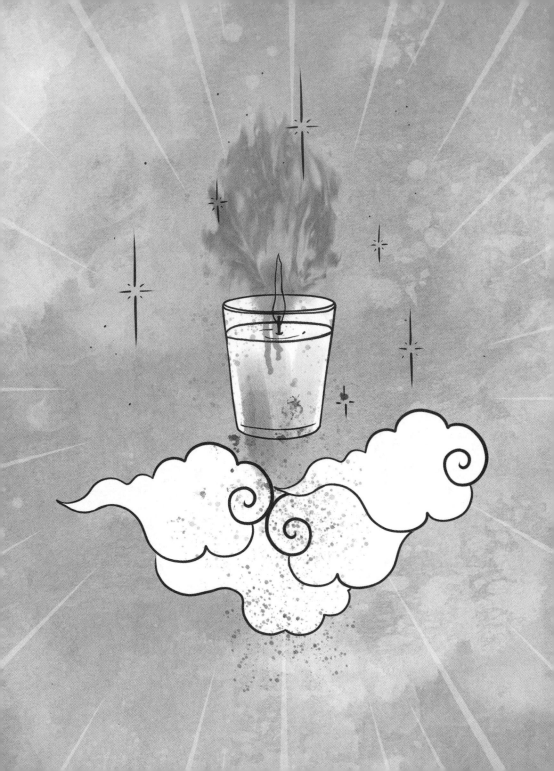

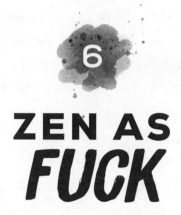

ZEN AS *FUCK*

> **"As a lamp in a windless place does not waver, so the transcendentalist, whose mind is controlled, remains always steady in his meditation on the transcendent self."**
> **—BHAGAVAD GITA 6.19**

At this point on our Rage Yoga journey, we have gathered all the tools to reach the summit. We have what we need to become Zen as fuck.

Okay, but what exactly does that mean?

Being Zen as Fuck

Being Zen as fuck means being aware of your mind, which gives you discipline in your thoughts. This gives you conscious control over your words and actions. When you are Zen as fuck, you don't live on autopilot, and you are almost magnetic. You draw a lot of Good Shit into your life in the form of great people and experiences. The unpredictability of circumstance and the waves of life don't easily rock you. Criticism, negativity, drama, and Bullshit don't touch you easily, and you're too busy being unapologetically awesome to seek validation from other people. Your connection to your Badass Self is so strong that outside influences have no real power over your confidence or happiness because you radiate these things from the inside out. Simply put, you're unfuckwithable.

The Bhagavad Gita is the Bible of traditional yoga. Much like you'd find in the Bible, in the Bhagavad Gita, you will find many grand stories that share teachings through metaphors. Sometimes their values are outdated, and the language they use to convey their message may be confusing (although, let's be real, a hell of a lot more proper than mine). Neither of these books are going to contain an excess of fuck words or analogies that include staring at ball sacks, but they do contain teachings similar to the ones that you'll find in this book. When it comes to being what I call "Zen as fuck," the Bhagavad Gita has a lot to say. One of my favorite passages about it is the one at the beginning of this chapter.

This passage really hits home the fact that yoga is a hell of a lot more than just physical postures. Beyond just getting flexible, strong, and improving your balance, yoga offers a workout for the mind. It's not just your willpower that starts to get rippling muscles; your entire brain gets jacked as fuck! As your mind becomes stronger, it becomes more resistant to the windstorms of life. The experience of being alive becomes a smoother one, because you don't find yourself getting whipped around as easily as a flame does when a breeze passes through. Doing the work means that this Zen as fuck state of mind steadily begins leaving the mat and coming with you into the rest of your life.

Regardless of whether or not you've totally absorbed all of what we've covered in the previous chapters, you deserve a supercharged high five! This shit is a lot, and you are clearly dedicated, you majestic badass! Kudos. You have the right to celebrate and give yourself a pat on the back. Take your time and do a happy dance, because you deserve it! I'll wait.

Are you dancing?

Are you done?

Because I have news:

The work isn't over.

I know! I am just *the fucking worst.*

Continuing Practice

Nothing is permanent. Being Zen as fuck doesn't mean that something has magically clicked inside you and now you'll be this way forever. No one is perfect, but you can find perfectly orgasmic sweet spots for moments at a time. It's a lot like doing a handstand. If you happen to be able to pull off a kick-ass handstand, kudos to you! Personally, I have been working on them for years. Although my handstand has gotten better over time, they require a lot of work, and I have to keep practicing.

You don't just miraculously balance in place for eternity when you do a handstand. You have to keep correcting and adjusting to stay balanced. The first thousand plus times you find that balance, even if only a split second, you see the matrix. It seems so simple all of a sudden, and you're almost surprised that getting there was ever a struggle. But inevitably, what goes up must come down! If you're dedicated to your practice, you keep at it and learn to find that sweet spot faster. You eventually stay there for longer periods of time. The corrections and adjustments start happening without much thought or effort. Still, even once they start to feel natural, you have to keep practicing. You can't just take a whole bunch of time off and then expect to be as adept when you come back to it. Your baseline might be higher than when you started the first time, but without dedication to your practice, things get rusty. Just like a balancing posture, maintaining a Zen as fuck life takes effort and willingness to continue doing the work.

BALANCING SEQUENCE

Find an unmoving point ahead of you to fix your gaze on. In traditional yoga this is called a *drishti*, and it helps with concentration as well as balance.

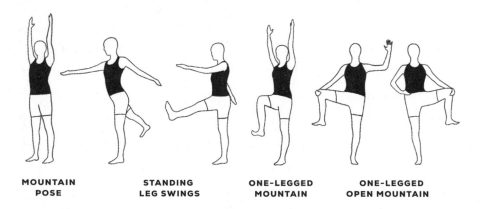

| MOUNTAIN POSE | STANDING LEG SWINGS | ONE-LEGGED MOUNTAIN | ONE-LEGGED OPEN MOUNTAIN |

Begin in a sturdy Mountain Pose at the front of your mat. Take five breaths here, exploring how your feet connect you to the ground and how your ankles support you. Perhaps experiment by lifting just your toes off of the mat. You can also try kicking your heels lightly inward while leaving them firmly planted on the ground. Notice how these adjustments change the engagement of your muscles, beginning in your feet and then up your legs and all throughout your body. Next, shift your weight, oh so slowly, into one foot. Let your raised foot begin to sway back and forth, gradually picking up speed and height as you begin Standing Leg Swings. While staying aware of your center of gravity, let your arms naturally swing to counterbalance your leg. Once you've found a comfortable rhythm, keep it up for five to seven breaths. Staying firmly grounded through your supporting leg, lift the other one as you come into One-Legged Mountain. As you stay here for three to five breaths, think about sending energy from your core, down through your supporting leg and through the entire bottom of your foot, to root you firmly into the ground. Bring your lifted leg out to the side, moving into One-Legged Open Mountain. Keep your focus on your unmoving point, or Drishti, and maintain that invisible root system from your core through to the ground. Stay here, you immovable badass, for three to five breaths.

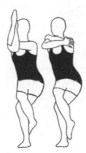

EAGLE POSE

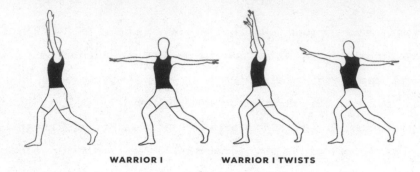

WARRIOR I　　　　**WARRIOR I TWISTS**

Keep your supporting leg rooted as you bring your raised leg down, crossing it over, coming into Eagle Pose. Lightly squeeze your legs together, combining their forces, so they can become one super leg. In whichever arm variation your prefer, squeeze your arms together, letting them become one super arm. Now you're full of super limbs! How's that going for you? Letting your inhales and exhales lift and anchor you, stay here for five breaths. Next, slowly unwind your limbs. Don't worry, you're still super! As your raised leg lifts off the supporting one, step it back and move into Warrior I. Breathe here, feeling your weight equally in both your legs and feet. Hold here for three breaths. Stay anchored down through your legs and feet as you begin Warrior I Twists. Move slowly. Only twist your upper body as far as you can without taking focus from the steadiness of your lower body. Twist each way three times then come back to your neutral starting position.

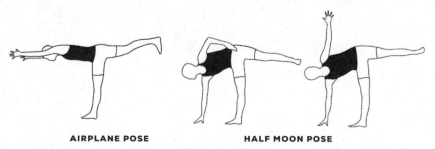

AIRPLANE POSE　　　　**HALF MOON POSE**

With your hands overhead, take a slight bend in your knees on your inhale. On your exhale, slowly lean your upper body forward as you shift your weight into your front foot. Stay aware (maybe even curious) as your back foot begins to take off, lifting you into Airplane Pose. Find your drishti, keep your supporting leg anchored as fuck, and breathe! Keep flying for three to five breaths. Like a martial artist in slow-motion, bring your arm from the same side of your body as your supporting leg down to the mat. Stay hella grounded in your supporting leg and powered up through your core as you begin to lift the other arm to the sky. As you do this, allow your body to open up the side. Welcome to Half Moon Pose, badass! Stay here for three to five breaths.

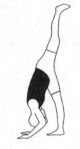

STANDING SPLIT

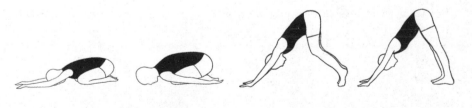

CHILD'S POSE   **DOWNWARD DOG**

Bring your lifted arm down to the mat to join the other and keep that incredibly grounding force coming on down through your supporting leg. Walk your hands closer to your foot and come into Standing Split. Take some weight into your hands as you take your lifted leg up higher and find some stillness here for three to five breaths. Next, bring your foot back down and let your body melt aaaalllllllll the way to the mat. Find yourself a comfortable Child's Pose and rest here for five breaths. When you're ready, move into Downward Dog. Find your foundation here, powering up from your core and down through your limbs. Take three steady breaths here.

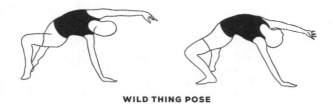

WILD THING POSE

Slowly lift one hand off of your mat. Keep on lifting that hand, reaching that arm up and over, beginning to open your body to the side. Engage your core, picking up the leg from the same side of your body as the reaching arm. Send that badass core strength through all your limbs, maintaining your balance, as your raised leg comes up and over, then steps down into Wild Thing Pose. Keep your foundation strong as you anchor yourself here, kicking ass for three to five breaths.

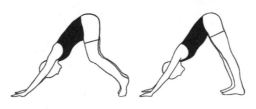

DOWNWARD DOG

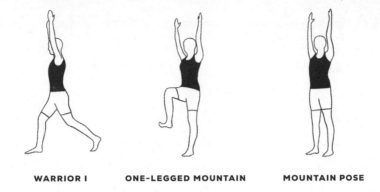

WARRIOR I   **ONE-LEGGED MOUNTAIN**   **MOUNTAIN POSE**

Keep steady in your breath as you flip back over to Downward Dog. Ground yourself here for three breaths. Next, inhale as you lift one leg back and up high behind you. Use you next exhale to supercharge your core, bringing your knee into your chest and stepping your foot forward. Stay rooted through your legs and come up onto your fingertips. Give yourself a slight push as you slowly stack your vertebrae, one at a time, rolling yourself up over your center of gravity and rising into a fierce-as-fuck Warrior I. Feel the strength in your legs and core, holding here for three breaths. Take a slight bend in your knees on your next inhale. On the following exhale, shift your weight into your front foot as you bring your back knee forward and up. Find your balance here in One-Legged Mountain Pose. Stay powered up in your core and down through your supporting leg. Kick butt (literally kicking invisible butts by extending your raised leg, if you feel so inclined) for three to five breaths. Slowly bring your raised foot down to the mat. Inhale your hands up overhead and exhale as you bring them down to the center of your chest. Finally, you majestic badass, give yourself a "fuck yeah!"

At this point, you might be wondering, *"If it's so much freakin' work and it doesn't just stick, why should I waste my time? This all sounds really boring, and I have a million better things to do, Lindsay! I have a life, you know. You're not my mom."*

You would be correct. I am not your mom.

I don't give a fuck if you've cleaned your room lately, but I am begging you to keep doing the work! Why begging, you ask? Maybe it's because I'm just selfish, but I desperately want to live in a world full of people who *actually* do the work. When someone finds that Badass Self and chooses to let it shine unapologetically, it makes a difference.

These people don't live life on autopilot. They become in touch with themselves and the world around them. This allows them to experience life through an authentic and empowered lens. Suddenly, their egos and happiness aren't easily affected by stupid shit because *they fucking love themselves.* By doing so, they rebel and weaken the social script. Rebels inspire rebellion, and holy shit, we need a rebellion! We need more people out there who are thinking and acting intentionally, not just reading their lines and playing an assigned role. These people can make things better (or even just a little less shitty) not just for themselves but for all of us. To put it quite simply, this world needs more majestic badasses and fewer giant assholes.

Sometimes doing the work really sucks. Looking into your darkness, challenging your fears, and calling out your own Bullshit isn't exactly a garden party. There are times it feels more like a bang-your-head-against-the-wall-and-scream party! Taking responsibility for yourself and your growth can be hard as hell, and that's why it can be tempting to avoid it.

This doesn't change the fact that the world needs fewer giant assholes, so put on your cape, you majestic badass! How's that for the world's worst sales pitch?

Imperfect Practice

Any activity that we enjoy because of how it engages our senses is what yoga often refers to as a "pleasure of the senses." Yoga teachings tell you to avoid the pleasures of the senses because they are distractions from enlightenment, which keep you from God. But unless you intend to live in an ashram or keep entirely away from society as we know it, abstaining completely isn't realistic for most of us.

We all have some choice pleasure-seeking activities in our lives. You could be into skydiving, roller derby, baking, photography, or Dungeons & Dragons. Many of our pastimes don't "cultivate a strong interpersonal or spiritual foundation" or whatever, at least not directly, but gosh they're fun! Or maybe you enjoy more risqué things like smoking, drinking, or real kinky adult stuff. There's a reason there are so many songs about sex, drugs, and rock and roll… Gosh *that shit is fuuuuuuun!*

Yoga says that "God is in everything." That greater something, or your ability to be your Badass Self, can be found in everything. As long as you're not hurting anyone or acting out of autopilot and you are honoring your Badass Self, then "un-yogic" things don't have to invalidate your entire practice. Practicing yoga doesn't mean you have to be perfect, and no one should be expected to be entirely wholesome. You can still enjoy sensory pleasures and have a good practice.

Sometimes indulging goes beyond fun, and these sensory pleasures can end up being used as crutches when someone is struggling. Leaning on overindulgent behavior is not an ideal coping mechanism, and it shouldn't be a go-to method of coping. But when it really comes down to it, there's nothing wrong with using a crutch as long as you're willing to learn to walk without it. Just don't let these things distract you so much that you stop practicing altogether.

I'm not endorsing addict behavior or saying that you should get lazy with your willpower muscle. Quite the opposite! People often overindulge to avoid their internal world and procrastinate on doing the kind of work necessary to step into their Badass Self. It's a tempting path because it looks like a super fun shortcut to happiness! But in the famous words of Admiral Ackbar, "It's a trap!" Avoiding and overindulging will only get in the way of being Zen as fuck. These paths are often taken out of fear, and the happiness they provide is painfully impermanent. Work that willpower muscle instead, and don't give up on your practice if that muscle gives in.

You will slip up from time to time, and you won't always be steady "like a lamp in a windless place." Curveballs and Bullshit are always going to be flying around unpredictably, and sometimes you're gonna get hit in the face. I don't know what to tell you; it's just going to happen. Expecting not to get hit would be like taking part in a water balloon fight and then being confused when you get wet. When you take a load to the face, it's okay to have feelings about it. It would be surprising if you didn't have feelings about it! It's normal to feel hurt, confused, or angry. It's okay to have uncomfortable or unsteady emotions. The part that matters most is what you do about them. We know that ignoring them, letting them mutate out of sight, is a bad idea. So how can you express and dismantle them constructively?

Getting Good at Stress

In case you haven't noticed, we don't live in a magical utopia. To put it lightly, the world that we live in can be *a tad* stressful. We might not actively seek stress out, and we can make choices to lessen it, but it will always be there in one way or another. So we might as well get good at it, right?

We all know the feeling of stress. It begins when the body releases adrenaline. Your heart starts pounding, and your senses become heightened, sometimes so much so that it feels unbearable! All the chatter in your head becomes white-hot noise, and you might even feel light-headed or start to shake. We've heard about the negative effects stress has on our hearts, that it restricts our blood vessels, increasing our chances of having a stroke and leading to high blood pressure. Rumors say it can even make us fat. We've been told often enough that stress is bad, for both our physical and mental health, that we've come to accept it as fact. However, it turns out this isn't necessarily true. Stress is not our enemy. In fact, sometimes it can be our friend.

The new science on stress is absolutely fascinating. It turns out that in stressful situations, our bodies don't just release adrenaline, they also release oxytocin. This hormone is partly responsible for making us feel happy. Have an orgasm? Oxytocin is there. Hug someone you love? Oxytocin. Pet a puppy? Oxy-totally-awesome-tocin. It might seem counterproductive that our bodies would release what we often refer to as a "happy hormone" when we're under stress, but it's brilliant. This is our bodies' way of taking care of themselves. In a way, they're looking out for us!

Oxytocin has some great benefits that help counteract the negative impact of stress. It physically strengthens your heart, which can heal previous damage and prevent more damage from happening in the future. Then it keeps encouraging you to reach out to your fellow humans for support. When you receive support, your body releases even more oxytocin. Bonus: it's *also* released when you give support to someone else. That's why it feels good to lift others up when they're down or to support a friend in need.* It also turns out that how you think about stress directly affects how your body responds to it. It can wreak havoc on your physical and mental state, but it doesn't have to. Your thoughts make all the difference. Our bodies are so connected to our minds that we have the power to use this connection to our advantage.

When you reframe your beliefs on the role of stress, you can change its physical effects. Instead of worrying about all the ways it can fuck you up, you can choose to view it as a positive thing. This isn't some "just think positive" bullshit. It's not about suppressing or denying how you feel when you experience stress. It's about acknowledging and accepting it. Instead of feeling like an overwhelmed meat puppet, you can use it as fuel. Whatever it is that is stressing you out, your body is giving you the energy and focus you need to rock the shit out of it. Your senses are kicking into high gear

---

* Unless of course this is someone who you've helped move, like, six times over the past two years, hauling their excessively large couch up three flights of stairs, all under a sense of obligation and the promise of pizza. But there never is pizza. Where is the pizza, Karen?!

so you can think clearly and decisively, and your blood is pumping faster to prepare you to be awesome. Whether you're breaking a sweat over a job interview or trembling in the wake of bad news, your stress response is preparing you to be courageous. Your biology is trying to help. When you think about this response as something that can benefit you, your blood vessels don't constrict, and your body can process the hormones that are flooding it without suffering damage. By practicing control over your thoughts and choosing an intentional response, you take away a lot of the power that stress has over you. You take that power as your own, stay in control of it, and learn to trust your Badass Self.

UJJAYI BREATH

Ujjayi Breath is often used to build a little extra "fire" when you need a boost of mental resilience. It can also give you a boost of extra strength and grit to push through physical challenges. Keep it in mind during difficult yoga sequences and poses! It warms your body up too; the "fire" part is no joke! This breath can even be used in cold environments to stay warm.

There are two common ways to cue this breath. One is to think about "smiling" in the back of your throat. The other is to think about holding an egg in your throat, which no one ever does, yet somehow this image works. Either way, you'll breathe in and out through your nose. Your inhale will be the same as usual. On your exhale, because of the peculiar shape this smile and/or egg has made in your throat, your breath will make a different sound than usual. If it's a little on the raspy side or if you sound like Darth Vader, then you're doing it right.

Repeat this. Inhale through your nose quietly, relaxing your body. Exhale through your nose while making this new weird shape in the back of your throat. Engage your abdominal muscles during your exhale to push air out of your lungs, making a sound like a Sith Lord.

Developing Power

You, my dear badass, hold a lot of power. As you move through this life, kicking ass and being Zen as fuck, remember this:

> **"WITH GREAT POWER COMES GREAT RESPONSIBILITY."**

Although most commonly associated with Uncle Ben from the universe of Spider-Man (thank you, Stan Lee), the origins of this quote are much harder to nail down than Spider-Man's. Winston Churchill, Theodore Roosevelt, and Voltaire are only some of the names that are often associated with this quote. There's a reason it has been said so many times through the ages...it's undeniably true! Radioactive blood or not, these words about power and responsibility still apply to you.

UNFUCKWITHABLE SEQUENCE

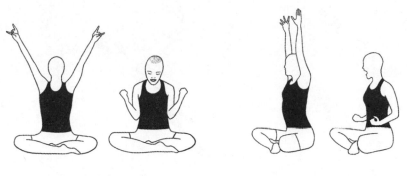

VICTORY BREATH

SEATED FISTS OF FIRE

From a cozy, seated position on your mat, begin with Victory Breaths. Open yourself up to all the Good Shit, soaking it in and basking in every inhale. Pull that Good Shit in as you compress with every exhale, squeezing out stale Bullshit. Once you've finished ten of these breaths, return to your neutral seated position and pause. Take a couple moments to ground yourself here and feel any new sensations that may be popping up throughout your body. You might feel warm and strong or light and relaxed. Take note! Next, begin Seated Fists of Fire. Lengthen your spine with your inhales. Get vocal and fire your core right the fuck up with every exhale. Keep it up for five to ten fiery breaths.

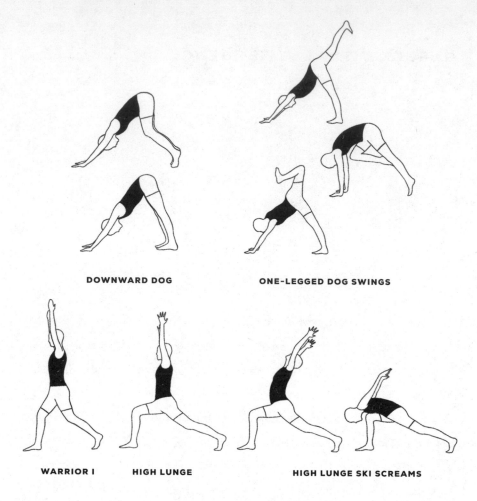

DOWNWARD DOG

ONE-LEGGED DOG SWINGS

WARRIOR I

HIGH LUNGE

HIGH LUNGE SKI SCREAMS

Moving into Downward Dog, send your energy from your core down through all of your limbs. Hold this pose for three breaths. Next, bring one leg up high behind you and begin One-Legged Dog Swings. Lift with your inhale, extending all the way through your raised heel. Fire up your core with your exhale, pulling your knee in toward your chest. Swing dat fine leg three to five times, then step your foot forward on your mat. Roll your body up one vertebrae at a time, rising like a mother fuckin' phoenix as you come into Warrior I. Take three breaths here, you majestic creature. Next, step your back foot farther to the back of your mat to come into High Lunge. Raise your arms over head as you inhale, expanding your chest and perhaps even arching backward slightly. Get loud with your next exhale as you begin High Lunge Ski Screams, staying grounded through your unshakable legs and core while your upper body folds down. Rise up again with your next inhale and repeat three to five times.

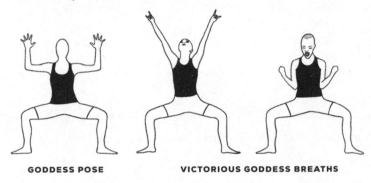

GODDESS POSE　　　　**VICTORIOUS GODDESS BREATHS**

Use the power of your next exhale to steady yourself, slowly pivoting on your feet to turn your body toward the open side of your mat. Feel your weight press down through your feet, evenly distributing through all parts of each sole, and bend your legs to come into Goddess Pose. Keep your spine tall and your shoulders engaged down your back as you open your arms wide. Feel your chest expand as your breath rolls up from your belly. Lift your chin, ready for anything, and stay here for three to five breaths. Inhale as you raise your hands up wide overhead and begin Victorious Goddess Breaths. Pull your elbows down into your sides with your exhales as your breath is forced out through your mouth. Inhale as you raise your arms again and repeat three to five times, using this breath to supercharge and reinforce your body and mind.

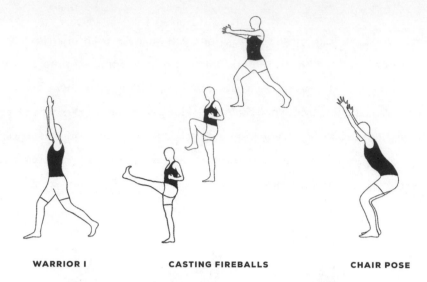

WARRIOR I   **CASTING FIREBALLS**   **CHAIR POSE**

Bring your arms overhead and, moving slow and steady, pivot on your feet to return to Warrior I. Take a slight bend in your legs and bring your arms forward to prepare for Casting Fireballs! Shift your weight into your front leg and bring your back knee forward, moving like the badass powerhouse that you are, while you pull your fists in beside your hips. Inhale to step your raised leg back and return your arms forward. Cast three to five more fireballs, then step your raised leg down. Bring your hands overhead and tap into your core as you sink down into Chair Pose, holding here for three to five breaths.

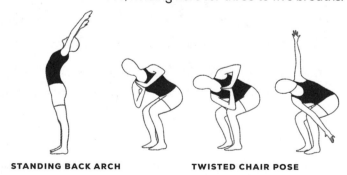

STANDING BACK ARCH   **TWISTED CHAIR POSE**

Rise back up into a standing position. Ground down through your fabulous legs as you move into Standing Back Arch. Use your inhales to lift and expand through your upper body as you ease into this back bend for three to five breaths. Release this posture as you sink your hips back down into Chair Pose before moving into Twisted Chair Pose. Stay steady and firm in your foundation as you get your twist on. Stay here for three to five breaths.

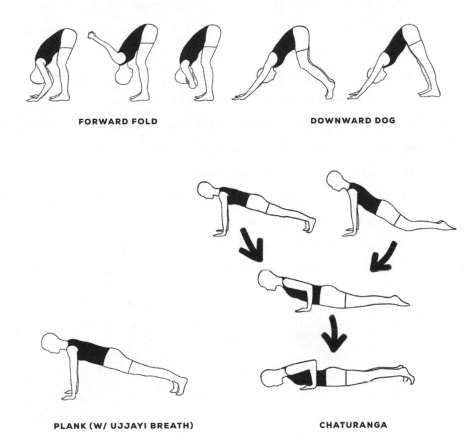

FORWARD FOLD

DOWNWARD DOG

PLANK (W/ UJJAYI BREATH)

CHATURANGA

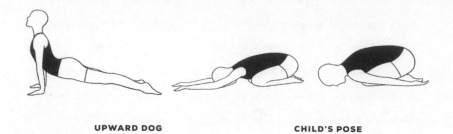

UPWARD DOG   **CHILD'S POSE**

Allow gravity to do its thing as you come into Forward Fold. Release your back muscles. Release your neck muscles. Just release! You deserve it. Take your time. Whenever you're ready, bring your hands to the mat and step back into Downward Dog. Spread your fingers wide, feeling each one pressing into the mat as you power up your arms and core. Use your Ujjayi Breath to supercharge your body while you shift your weight into your hands and begin moving into Plank Pose. Lower down into Chaturanga while you continue to stoke the fiery force of your breath, letting its strength move through your body. Maintain this whole-body-badass engagement and press into your hands as you lift into Upward Dog. Marinate in the merriment of this posture, allowing your chest to expand and your chin to lift. At your leisure, in any way you damn well please, come into Child's Pose. Rest.

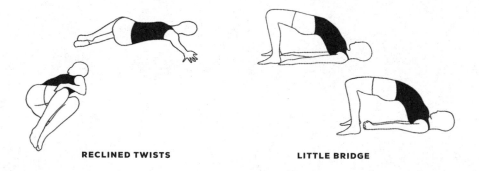

RECLINED TWISTS   **LITTLE BRIDGE**

Carry on this restful goodness as you find your way onto your back. Let your upper body melt into your mat as you come into Reclined Spinal Twist. Inhale the Good Shit and exhale the Bullshit, staying here for five to ten breaths before getting your Reclined Spinal Twist on in the other direction. Once you feel sufficiently twisted, place your feet flat on your mat and lift your hips up into Little Bridge. Picture the ground supporting you and pushing back as you press into it. You and the ground make a fantastic team! You also make an indestructible bridge. Lift, ground, and be badass for five to ten breaths.

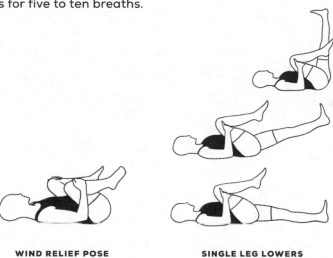

WIND RELIEF POSE   **SINGLE LEG LOWERS**

Lower your hips and pull your knees into your chest as you come into Wind Relief Pose. Feel your abdomen expand and press into your legs, giving you a gentle massage while your breath comes in and goes out. In your private bubble of calm, revel in stillness here for as long as you like. Release one knee and straighten this leg upward as you come into Single Leg Lowers. As it slowly descends to your mat, imagine sending active energy up and out through your heel. Use your core to elongate your torso, firmly flatten-ing your back to the mat, and continue pulling your other knee into your body. Once your leg reaches the mat, pull that knee into your body, then complete this movement with your other leg.

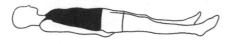

HAPPY ADULT NAP TIME

Extend both legs on your mat. Picture yourself creating an unfuckwithable force field as you connect with your breath. Close your eyes. Happy Adult Nap Time.

The practices and philosophies used in this book are not new. They have been around for a long time, in different forms and methodologies, to help people connect to something bigger. Call it God, or the Universe, or a Higher Power, or call it Snowball! Personally, I still prefer Badass Self. Whatever your spiritual beliefs may or may not be, you cannot deny the potential power of a mind that is fine-tuned and focused. When you follow these practices and philosophies, your mind can become just that! Some people may stumble into powerful roles by chance through the social script (hooray, classism and nepotism!) but anyone can develop some level of power. The question is then what do you do with it?

Siddhis

Traditional yoga says that someone who develops a deep connection to God will be so in touch with the ethereal material that comprises the universe that they can develop powers, called *siddhis*. These powers can be anything from telepathy to the ability to levitate. The same teachings also warn practitioners that should they receive these powers, they should not use them. They say that many well-practiced Yogis have been tempted by siddhis and that the ones who use it end up on a very different—and very dark—path.

We can all think of situations where people use their power in shitty ways. We can recount way the hell too many stories of people in positions of authority who have used that authority to abuse those with less. We can think of cult leaders brainwashing their devoted followers, stealing their income or leading them to mass suicide. Or how about sentient cheese puffs with toupees, spitting gasoline and throwing matches on a global scale?! There is no question about it: power in the wrong hands is dangerous.

Your Power

Outside a magic show, you likely haven't seen anyone levitate lately. I haven't seen it myself, but in this wild-ass time we live in, I feel like I've seen even wilder shit happen. No, I don't think that you're going to start shooting webs from your wrists (at least not by practicing yoga). Nothing is impossible, but I'd still say it's highly unlikely. You are, however, *very fucking likely* to develop power.

This internal practice can turn you into a confident free thinker with a steady mind, and this makes you magnetic. When those who are magnetic make themselves heard, they develop influence. If influence is given direction, it becomes power. This process could be reduced to something like a mathematical formula with variables. These variables can be altered to achieve a desired outcome. Depending on where you focus your mind and where you then choose to direct your influence, you can get many different results.

CONFIDENT FREE THINKER (X FOCUS) + STEADY MIND (X FOCUS) = MAGNETIC PERSON

MAGNETIC PERSON + BEING HEARD = INFLUENCE

INFLUENCE + DIRECTION = POWER

If you do the work to cultivate a Zen as fuck life and mindset, that will be your focus. You'll continue your practice, growing as a confident free thinker and strengthening your steady mind. When these two qualities are mixed and united under a shared focus, they can turn you into a magnetic person. Magnetic people have an easy time drawing the experiences and people that align with their focus into their lives. This might sound like "some hippie shit" with no tangible value, but it has real impact.

Magnetic people create their own badass reality, affecting the world around them. They leave impressions upon others by poking holes in societal scripts and breaking free of Bullshit cycles. This lessens the grip that scripts and cycles have on the here and now, as well as the grip they could have on future generations. We need more people who love themselves and inspire others to do the same. We need badasses, who are vulnerable enough to be courageous, connecting and caring for people instead of building walls between them. Can we get more people actively dismantling their anger and fear, neutralizing its poison, and using it as fuel to make things better? Can we get more of these magnetic people, please?

Zen as Fuck Revolution

Newton's third law of motion states that every action has an equal and opposite reaction. A force pushing one way will be met by an equally strong force pushing right back at it. Beyond just physical force, traditional yogic teachings apply this to emotional and energetic forces as well. It's a very simple way of describing a complex issue that you can see at play in all conflict, from a passive-aggressive fight between roommates to deadly global wars. Because of this, yoga teaches passivity. It says that kindness, patience, and compassion are the only things that can defuse things like corruption, violence, or injustice.

It's a complex world we're living in. It's constantly changing, and as it does, sometimes our beliefs and practices need to adapt as well. Traditional teachings are right in saying that force is met with force. It's true that kindness, patience, and compassion can defuse an opposing force. But if you pair these things with passive nonaction, you'll likely only be a door-mat. Somewhere in between passive nonaction and violent force, there is another answer. There is an argument to be made for the constructive use of power. It can be used responsibly to create your individual badass real-ity and, on a larger scale, to make our shared reality a more badass one. Honestly, that shared reality could use some help.

Power is used irresponsibly all the time. There are too many people with excessive power who don't have compassion and empathy to balance it out. They're so motivated by greed that they have selfishly devastated the environment to a point where our very future is endangered. They benefit by using people like puppets, turning them against one another, and per-petuating racist and classist systems. These assholes benefit from our fear and take advantage of passive nonaction.

You're allowed to be angry.

In fact, *we all should be in a fucking rage!*

But what are we going to do with that rage?

Passive nonaction won't change shit. To see any change, especially on the larger stages of the world, people have to make themselves heard. They should act intentionally from a place of courageous vulnerability. They need to be steady in conflict, allowing them to harness the strength of their rage to affect real change instead of causing extreme forces to push back. These people need to show up and do the work, not just on these larger stages but in their personal lives as well, so they can remain kind, patient, and com-passionate. This work will help keep their egos in check, allowing them to avoid the traps of power so they can continue to use that power responsibly.

The world will benefit from you leading a Zen as fuck life. Being unapologetically awesome and authentically fearless will always make a difference. It's a simple yet bold rebellion.

So, you majestic badass...

Welcome to the revolution.

Rage on!

Can I get a "Fuck yeah!"?

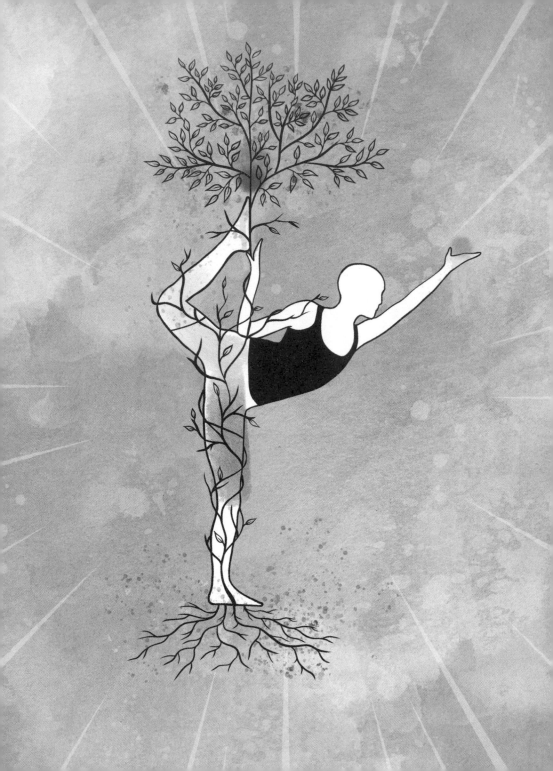

CREATING
A REGULAR
PRACTICE

Enthusiasm and inspiration are great. You can use those things as fuel to keep you motoring along, but they aren't reliable. The tide comes in, and the tide goes out; it's never permanently fixed in one place. If you really want to have a successful practice, the best way to make sure that it sticks is to turn it into a reliable and disciplined habit. Here are some tips and tricks that you can use to take these lessons and turn them into awesome habits for optimal ass kicking.

Set Goals and Make a Plan

The first step is to set some goals. What is it you want to achieve from your practice? Are there specific mental, emotional, physical, or spiritual benefits that you would like to experience? What does it look and feel like to you? Once you have this destination in mind, you'll need to chart yourself a course to get there. Otherwise, you'll be wandering around all willy-nilly. Charting your course means that it's time to make a map or a step-by-step plan that will lay out how you will reach your goals.

You'll want to look at your goals realistically and think about all the steps necessary to get from where you are now to where you want to be. This book will have already given you some methods to help you get there, and you might even have some preexisting knowledge in your arsenal already. Fucking awesome! Which methods will be useful for your particular goals? How can you use all these different tools and techniques as steps along your path?

Remove Barriers

What is standing in between you and your practice goals? This can be a surprisingly difficult question to answer. On the surface, it seems simple, but sometimes you need to ask the question several times and take a ruthless magnifying glass to yourself to find the barriers. The answers may not be obvious at first. Keep a careful watch on your habits, and you may find some interesting answers.

Barrier: Knowledge Gaps

Are you holding back because there are gaps in the path you've charted toward your goals? If so, cut that shit out! Get out of your head, get your head out of your ass, and don't let yourself get paralyzed by overthinking it. You're going to discover more questions on the way, so how could you possibly be expected to have all the answers right fucking now? You can always search for the answers to your questions by finding a teacher or doing some research. If you wait for all the answers and for perfect conditions, you may never get going. Be ready to learn and trust that you will fill the gaps in as you go. Just. Start.

Barrier: Lack of Time

Look, I'm not going to pretend I know exactly what is going on in your life. However, I do know that this is an excuse and not actually a barrier. I get it! You're busy. We all are. Still, as busy as we might be, time is a nonrenewable resource that we constantly spend. Instead of thinking you lack time, ask yourself how you're spending it. Rather than saying "I don't have time," start watching how you prioritize it. If it's actually a priority for you, you'll manage to find the time in your schedule. Some of the things you choose to spend your time on can be limited, delegated, or cut out completely. You have time for a yoga practice; you just may need better time management skills. Even a short five-minute practice is infinitely better than a zero-minute one.

Barrier: Lack of Space

Just as with time, if it's a priority, you will find space. Many people overestimate how much room they actually need for an at-home physical practice. Just a couple of feet of open space can be used, even if you're cramped in a tiny apartment. Trust me, I would know! Alternatively, you can go outside, to a studio, or to a friend's house. Maybe you just need to reorganize and downsize your shit!

Bonus: many of those off-mat practices take zero space.

If it's a quiet at-home space you lack, you can still find a work-around. Some of my favorite strategies include sharpening your ability to focus in noisy environments, laying down boundaries with others for your practice time, or finding a different space altogether. The "I don't give a fuck what other people think" strategy will also increase your options of spaces where you can practice.

Barrier: Lack of Proper Equipment

You don't need expensive clothing or fancy equipment. No bells, whistles, gongs, or panpipes necessary. You just need a body. BOOM! Barrier removed.

Barrier: Not in Good Enough Shape

Bullshit! This is like saying you can't take your car to a car wash because it's too dirty. Getting in better physical shape is one of the top reasons people begin practicing yoga. If you're going to classes in a studio that do not feel inclusive for your skill level or for your body, try a different class. Maybe even try a different studio. If you prefer, a solid at-home practice means only your plants can see you! Plants tend to leaf judgment out of it anyway. They're rooting for you. There are plenty of awesome resources you can use to find what you need, both online and in books *ahem*. If the poses and sequences in these resources don't fit your needs, try finding some new ones! There are a lot of options out there.

Customize

Remember, this is *your* practice. That means you get to do whatever the fuck you want. You get to choose what your practice looks like, and you don't have to follow someone else's rules. It can be as long or as short as you want, and it can happen as frequently as you like. You don't have to hit the mat for five hours every fucking day for it to be a real and valid practice! The chances are that you'll find your own rhythm over time, and as long as you put real energy into it, your practice will be great.

Make Rituals

When you brush your teeth before bed, that is part of a ritual. If you're one of those people who never steps on a sidewalk crack, there's an element of ritual to that. Some people can't even imagine the mornings without their coffee, and others can't comprehend an evening without TV. There are many rituals we partake in all the time without even realizing it, and it feels weird if we don't do them. Our brains are really just glorified supercomputers, so when we do anything regularly enough, it recognizes those activities as patterns and begins to anticipate them. Brains, just like computers, really like to assume "if X, then Y." You can use this to your advantage by creating rituals around the habits you want to develop. It's like coding your own brain!

Since they're how we form our experiences, senses are a major contributing factor to how we form habits. Adding an extra sensory component into the habits that you're trying to form makes them more likely to get hardwired in. We have five senses: taste, touch, smell, hearing, and sight. If you get creative, you can find some ways to add them into your formula.

Every time I sit to write this book, I apply some essential oils and look at a dorky inspirational poster that I made.* I make coffee, turn on the lamp at my desk, put on my fuck-off headphones, and then I get started. Even though I'm not someone who focuses easily, this works really well for me. I've trained my brain to correlate the smell of orange oil with focusing. I see the dorky inspirational poster, taste the coffee, touch the lamp's switch, and hear the music. All these things have been hardwired in as cues for me now. When I experience them, my brain kicks into gear and is ready to kick ass.

It can also help to have rituals and habits around ending your practice. This will help your mind prepare to move back into the day-to-day world. A really great example of this is shavasana, otherwise known as Corpse Pose (or, by me, Happy Adult Nap Time). Shavasana is massively beneficial right after a physical practice! It will help the benefits and experience points you've just earned on the mat settle into your body and mind. It will help your balance improve more quickly, your muscles repair faster, and any personal insights you had stick.

A closing ritual teaches your brain that what you were doing is now a complete, neatly wrapped-up event. Now that this process has a distinct

---

* This poster includes some cheesy uplifting quotes and some photos that inspire me. There's a photo of someone working away at their desk, looking chill as fuck, with balanced scales in the background. There's a picture of a happy author holding a physical copy of their new book. There is also one of Angelina Jolie as Lara Croft from *Lara Croft: Tomb Raider*, because she's a decisive and efficient badass. We could all stand to be more like Lara Croft!

end, you're wonderful computer of a brain will have an easier time hard-wiring this pattern in. Also, since it signifies the definite end of an event, a closing ritual can help you move from one finished activity into the rest of your day with more ease. Which rituals can you use to hardwire your practice into a habit? Can you think of ways to incorporate your senses into them?

Improvise and Adapt

As you venture out to crush your goals, you may find that things shift. Sometimes a course gets altered and goals get reprioritized. As you grow and change, these things will do the same. It'd be really weird if they didn't. Just in case you need to be reminded, you're an adult, dammit! You're allowed to change your mind, and you don't need permission to do so. Take the wheel, Captain Badass.

If you build a badass practice but find it slipping, don't worry. You're not alone! Sometimes, no matter how much ass you kick, shit happens. You get sick, or something happens at work, or you end up moving, adopting a dog, get thrown off by holiday plans, etc. It happens! Hold yourself accountable, but don't crucify yourself. In the meantime, while conditions are not so ideal, don't give up! Be a chameleon and adapt.

Perhaps, due to unforeseen circumstances, you find yourself with less available time than usual. Try practicing for less time, even if only for five minutes! It can also help to check in (again) with how you are spending your time. It might be an easy mental break to dick around on your cell phone for a couple of minutes, but a short practice would be more beneficial. If you catch yourself opening up that app that you know you spend too much time on, stop, drop, and yoga!

If you're having a hard time getting on the mat, adapt by incorporating some more off-mat practices. We've covered quite a few throughout this book. The great thing about these practices is that they don't have to take up a lot of time or space. Most of them are also very easy to incorporate in your day-to-day life! While these practices are always best done with full focus, many of them can be done while you're doing other things. This could mean repeating mantras or affirmations while in the shower or waiting in line. It could be doing breath work while you're folding laundry or washing the dishes. Pick a couple of favorites, and get them in your day.

You can also do what I like to call "fidget practice." Sneak in tiny bits throughout the day in the gaps of time that you usually spend just fidgeting between activities. What're you doing? Waiting for the coffee to brew, the toast to pop, or your ride to arrive? You can get some stealthy practice in during these times, and it will be much more beneficial than just standing around and fidgeting. You can bust out a couple of basic postures, breathe, and recenter yourself. This time can also easily be filled with off-mat practices. If you find yourself in a busy atmosphere and feel self-conscious about doing anything too physical, you can swap in these practices without drawing much unwanted attention.

If you're trying to keep a low profile, you could try off-mat practices such as cyclical breaths, ksepana mudra, uttarabodhi mudra, or internal repeating of mantras or affirmations. For physical practices, you can try One-Legged Mountain Pose or Standing Leg Swings. You can keep these poses extra low profile by shifting your weight and just baaaaaaarely moving your lifted leg. Some postures, like Cat-Cow, Reclined Figure 4, and Seated Spinal Twist, can even be done from a seated position at your desk.

If you're not too worried about drawing some attention to yourself, you can squeeze in some off-mat practice with Ujjayi Breath, Let That Shit Go Breath, Kapalabhati Breath, or vocal repeating of mantras or affirmations. For physical practices, you can try Goddess Flows, Warrior II Flows, or Seated Flows, or you can string a couple of poses together to create a short flow of your own. You can also bust out a brief intuitive movement practice or practice a single posture. My favorite postures to do on their own include Downward Dog, Bob's Cosmic Dancer, Cat-Cow, Party People, and One-Legged Mountain.

Feed Your Fire

Motivation and inspiration are fucking rocket fuel, but they can be fickle fuckers. You can't always count on them to be there. However, there are some things you can do to encourage them to stick around longer and come by more often. This is another opportunity to hack into the mainframe of your computer brain to customize the programming for optimal awesome.

When I binge-watched nine seasons of *RuPaul's Drag Race*, it infiltrated the way I spoke, and my fashion sense became a little "extra." When I started listening to a podcast about how law intersects with philosophy and today's social issues, I found I started talking a bit lawyer-y. I started debating both sides of silly things like the merits of wetting your toothbrush before or after applying toothpaste.

Whatever you take in through your senses stays in the forefront of your mind and starts expressing itself through you. It's important to be cognizant of what you're consuming and how it comes out because this really takes the expression "you are what you eat" to the next level! If you want to stay motivated and inspired in your practice, go out of your way to find stuff related to it: podcasts, communities, blogs, movies, art, books, etc. Let your mind ingest it the way your body ingests vitamins. It will help your relationship with inspiration and motivation stay strong and healthy.

Just Fucking Do It

The simplest yet most crucial tip for building a badass practice is this:

JUST. FUCKING. DO. IT.

Feel a bit stiff today? Short on time? Something unexpected happened? Do it anyway, even if it means customizing or adapting your practice. Not seeing the physical results you wanted? Feeling more like a caffeinated squirrel than a Zen as fuck badass? Keep going!

Inspired by the ideas of Aristotle, Will Durant said, "We are what we repeatedly do. Excellence, then, is not an act, but a habit." If you continuously make excuses and repeatedly half-ass your efforts, that is the habit you're setting yourself up for. If you keep moving forward, even in the face of obstacles, you're creating the habit of being an ass kicker. Even if sometimes that means moving as slow as a turtle crawling through peanut butter, any forward momentum is better than no momentum! Just keep putting one foot in front of the other. It's as simple as that.

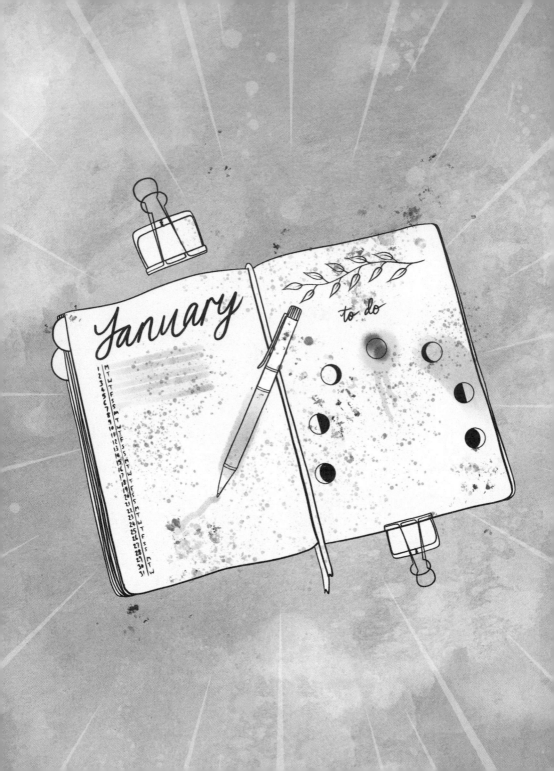

8

SEVEN-DAY
RAGE YOGA
PROGRAM

What with all the poop jokes, rants about weird circus shit, and all the movement and practices we've played with, I hope you've had fun! Still, I imagine that you haven't read all the way through this book just for funsies, right? You got this far because you want to build your own badass practice and lead that Zen as fuck life. To make it happen, you've equipped yourself with tools and knowledge.

Knowledge is power. That's great and all, but that power is useless unless it's applied. If you're sending a package through the mail but you never apply a postage stamp to it, it's going nowhere. We also don't really have an embodied understanding of our knowledge until we put it into action. If you apply a stamp to that same package but it never leaves your kitchen table, it's *still* useless *(except maybe as a paperweight)*. Effective learning doesn't come from just reading or listening to people talk about things. On average, after twenty-four hours, people only retain about 10 percent of the information they read. But we do retain about 75 percent if we put that information into action. So, badass, let's fucking do this!

In this seven-day Rage Yoga program, you'll find that each day has three sections.

1. **Theme:** When you first read the theme, take a couple of minutes to think about it and let it soak in. Use this as a sort of filter to experience your day through. Revisit the theme before you do your movement sequence, at least once during your day, and then again before bed.

2. **Breath Practice and Movement Sequence:** Every day, there is a breath to practice as well as a movement sequence. These are separate things! Don't get me wrong, I really do hope that you're breathing throughout the sequence, but it's important to practice the breath by itself as well. Before you start your sequence, or even at a completely separate time, do your breath work, and then sit for a short while before moving on. This stillness after is meant to give you time to check in with your mind and body, to notice any new thoughts or sensations, and to let the experience points sink in.

3. **Homework:** Your homework will be one extra tidbit of goodness to boost your practice. It might look like another breath practice, a thought exercise, or a meditation. This homework can be done in conjunction with the other daily program pieces

or by itself. Keep your theme in mind when doing your homework. I highly recommend journaling about your experiences! You'll be likely to make some interesting discoveries and have an easier time processing them think-y parts.

DAY 1: CUT YOURSELF SOME SLACK

Theme: As you start out today, you have one goal—cut yourself some slack! Allow yourself to make mistakes and to be imperfect. Learning is a wonderfully messy process, and so is life! Fuck! Expecting perfection from yourself is unfair. Cut yourself some slack both on and off your mat. If you catch your inner voice starting to be a jerk, take a second. Pause. Inhale the Good Shit. Exhale the Bullshit. And move on!

Breath Practice and Movement Sequence: Inhale Good Shit and Exhale Bullshit (chapter 1), Breath and Movement Sequence (chapter 1).

Homework: Read the "Learn, Trust, and Look Foolish" section in chapter 5, under the heading "Creating Your Badass Reality." If you falter during your movement sequence or slip up doing day-to-day stuff, shrug it off (maybe even with a smile).

DAY 2: LET THAT SHIT GO

Theme: We all have baggage and anxieties that like to pop up and be assholes. These assholes can take many forms. See if you can spot the

Bullshit that is clinging on to you and take steps toward letting it go. This often means forgiving yourself and others. Be it from a misunderstanding, a mistake, or intentional harm, our past experiences can really sink their hooks into us. Letting go and/or mustering true forgiveness isn't always easy. Sometimes it doesn't even feel possible! If you're grappling with some particularly sticky Bullshit, try reframing "letting go" as "loosening the grip." Remember, this grip goes both ways! Your baggage holds on to you, but you also hold on to it. Struggling to let go doesn't mean that you're fucked up or weak. It means that you got through some rough crap and it left a mark. You made it through. You did good.

Breath Practice and Movement Sequence: Let That Shit Go Breath (chapter 1), Letting Go Sequence (chapter 1).

Homework: Kapalabhati Breath (chapter 1).

 # DAY 3: INTUITION

Theme: You are wiser and stronger than you know. Trust yourself! If you find that you doubt yourself or your abilities today, your mission is to first give yourself a high five for catching the thought, then do a quick posture check and repeat a mantra or affirmation that makes you feel like the majestic badass that you are. Try the affirmation "I am enough. I am worthy," or look up some inspiration in chapter 3 for something that feel right to you.

Breath Practice and Movement Sequence: Ujjayi Breath (chapter 6), Intuitive Sequence (chapter 3).

Homework: Posture vs. Thought Experiment (chapter 2).

DAY 4: UNAPOLOGETICALLY AWESOME

Theme: Today your mission is to let your Badass Self shine! Don't wait for permission to be yourself or for validation to see your own worth. Lean in to the things that make you feel good, perhaps even euphoric. Follow those feelings instead of letting discomfort or fear be your main guiding force.

Breath Practice and Movement Sequence: Let That Shit Go Breath (chapter 1), Unapologetically Awesome Sequence (chapter 5).

Homework: Unapologetically Awesome Reality Check (chapter 4).

DAY 5: HERE. NOW.

Theme: Your mission today is to spend as much time as you can coming from an intentional place. Stay as mindful as you can in your mind and body. Watch your thoughts, words, and actions. Ask yourself what purpose they are serving and if that purpose best serves you. It's normal to spend time living in autopilot mode, so don't worry. No one is expecting you to be mindful and intentional every second of the day! Do what you can, and if you wanna go the extra mile, journal about your experience with this today. Note how much time you spend on autopilot and what your autopilot behaviors are. How would you like them to be in the future?

Breath Practice and Movement Sequence: Cyclical Breath (chapter 1), Slow Down Sequence (chapter 2).

Homework: Thought Observation Meditation (chapter 2).

DAY 6: FEARLESS FREAK

Theme: Whaddya want? This isn't about what other people want, what they might want for you, or whatever is easiest. This is about what *you* want. What would you aim for, in both your present and future life, if fear was not a problem? Today, your mission is to ask this question and let it simmer. You might not have a solid answer by the end of the day. Take your time! Whenever it comes to you, write your answer down, and keep it somewhere safe.

Breath Practice and Movement Sequence: Kapalabhati Breath (chapter 1), Fearless Sequence (chapter 5).

Homework: Dismantle Your Fear (chapter 5).

DAY 7: UNFUCKWITHABLE

Theme: Today's mission is to be steady, "like a flame in a windless place." To do this, you'll need to use the key takeaways from all the previous days. You'll need to cut yourself slack, let go, trust yourself, be present, and be fearless. That's a lot of stuff, but when you put it all together, you carry a hella lotta power! Even if it's only for moments at a time, you'll know when you hit all those targets at once. You'll be unfuckwithable. You'll be Zen as fuck!

Breath Practice and Movement Sequence: Ujjayi Breath (chapter 6), Unfuckwithable Sequence (chapter 6).

Homework: Read the section "Getting Good At Stress" (chapter 6). Hold this in mind if/when your day gets stressful.

GLOSSARY OF POSES

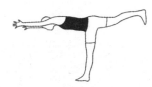

AIRPLANE POSE

How-To: Begin in a standing position with your arms overhead. Shift your weight onto one foot as you lift the other. Keep your core engaged, bringing the lifted leg behind you. Allow your upper body to bend forward with your arms outstretched as your back leg extends straight behind you, finding a strong and connected line from your wrists to your back heel. Woo! You're an airplane!

Tips: Keeping your back leg engaged with your foot flexed will help in finding balance. Making airplane noises never hurts either. Avoid letting your body twist open to the side.

Transitions: This pose is often transitioned to/from Mountain Pose, High Lunge, and Warrior I. A less common (and super fancy) transitional pose is Standing Split.

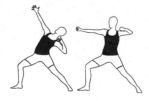

ARCHER RELEASE

How-To: Start off in Warrior II. Next, move your arms into a position as though you are holding a bow. Load that invisible bow with whatever emotional or mental stuff that you want to let go of. Lock, load, and get ready! When you release your arrow, sending that Bullshit off into the abyss and far away from your Badass Self, lean your upper body toward your back foot to come into a side bend. Stay lengthened through your spine and allow this bend to come from your waist. Once done, reset into your starting position.

Tips: Engage your core to lift and lengthen your upper body as you lean into your side bend, moving as though you have a wall directly in front of your chest and another behind your back. Avoid turning your chest forward and coming into a back bend.

Transitions: Archer Release can be a great transition into Exalted Warrior or, if you cartwheel your hands forward, High Lunge with hands on the mat.

BAD PONY

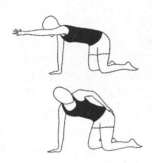

How-To: Get yourself into a position on all fours. Inhale as you lift one arm forward, parallel to the ground. Exhale as you bring that hand back towards your fine booty and give it an appreciative tap. As you reach back, let your gaze follow your fingers to stretch and wake up the side of your body. On your following inhale, reach forward again. Repeat this motion for several breaths, giving that bad pony a little smack on your exhale and reaching forward with your inhale.

Tips: Keep your core engaged to avoid arching your back. Arching will cheat you out of a good side stretch.

Transitions: Cat-Cow or Mother Fuckin' Unicorn are great follow up poses. Bad Pony can also be transitioned through Child's Pose or Downward Dog.

BANANA POSE

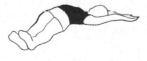

How-To: Lay on your back and reach your arms overhead. Slowly inch your feet and upper body towards one side of the mat, keeping your hips in one place, until your body comes into a banana-like shape. Breathe deeply and relax into this posture, finding a deliciously aPEELing side body stretch.

Tips: Don't rush this pose! Focus on how the sensations of the stretch change as your breath comes and goes.

Transitions: Banana Pose is great to put near the end of your sequence because it's a very relaxing posture. Try transitioning to it from Reclined Twists or to lowering to it from Boat Pose.

BOAT POSE

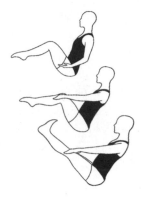

How-To: Sitting on your booty, bend your legs with your knees together and feet planted flat. Lean back until your core engages, lengthening your spine and straightening your lower vertebrae. Keep leaning back and engaging that kick-ass core as you slowly lift your feet off the mat. You can leave your fingertips of the mat to help you balance or kick it up a notch by bringing your arms in front of you and parallel to the mat. As you get more comfortable, try lifting your legs higher and begin to straighten them.

Tips: Avoid curving your back by engaging your core and keeping your spine tall as fuck. This "tall as fuck" engagement goes right from your tailbone and up through your neck.

Transitions: You can rock your boat back then forward to bring yourself onto your feet. From here you can transition to Downward Dog or Mountain Pose. Alternatively, you can lower yourself to your back for Banana Pose or Happy Adult Nap Time.

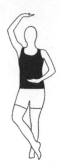

BOB'S COSMIC DANCER

How-To: Begin standing and shift your weight onto one foot, lifting the other. Cross the lifted ankle in front of the supporting one. Turn your lifted knee out by engaging and rotating from your hip. Whichever leg is crossed over, move your arm from the opposite side of your body overhead as if to press away from the ceiling. Move your other arm as if pressing away from the floor. Feel like getting extra jazzy? Play with the position of your arms, alternating them up, down, and out to the sides as you stay grounded through your supporting leg, maintaining your majestic dancer-like posture.

Tips: Maintain active engagement throughout your body by imagining you are pulling energy through the ground. Picture it coming up through your legs, into your torso, and then out through your fingertips and head. Avoid letting your shoulders roll forward.

Transitions: Bob's Cosmic Dancer is easily entered through Mountain Pose. It can also be a great transition into Warrior II by sweeping back the lifted leg.

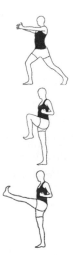

CASTING FIREBALLS

How-To: Starting in Warrior I, take both of your hands forward with your wrists together and palms open forward like your casting a sweet fireball! Take an inhale here, bending your legs slightly. Next, exhale sharply through your mouth, bringing your back knee forward and up like you're kneeing someone in the groin. As you do this, curl your hands into fists and pull them to the sides of your hips. Step back on the inhale and ready your hands to cast another fireball. If it feels good, put some extra force behind your exhale. Get fucking loud! Repeat several times.

Tips: Pick a fixed point to stare at while doing this. It will help you balance! Casting Fireballs will be more challenging the farther you step back on your inhales.

Transitions: If you hold the one-legged position on your exhale, this can be a great transition into One-Legged Mountain, Eagle Pose, or Airplane Pose.

CAT-COW

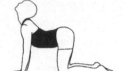

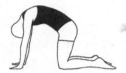

How-To: Start in a position on all fours. Exhale into Cat by rounding your back, just like a pissed off kitty. Next, inhale to Cow by arching your back, dropping your belly button down and sending your gaze upwards. Alternate back and forth between these two positions.

Tips: In Cat, get deep into your neck and shoulders by sending your gaze to your belly button and engaging your core. As you alternate between these postures, focus on the sensation and connecting your breath to your movement. Don't worry about achieving an "ideal" shape with your body. Cats and cows don't give a shit about shapes, they just do what feel good!

Transitions: Downward Dog or Child's Pose are common transitional poses to move into and out of Cat-Cow. Piss On Everything compliments this one well too.

CHAIR POSE

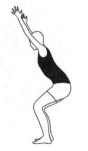

How-To: Begin standing with your arms up overhead. On your exhale, slowly bend your knees while keeping them stacked over your ankles. As your body sinks down, let your hips move back, keeping your lower body grounded. Using the engagement of your core, lengthen and lift your upper body. Maintain a strong line from your tailbone and up through your neck. If you kind of look like someone who is freaked out about sitting down in a portable toilet, then... you're probably doing it right.

Tips: Make sure you can see your toes as you sink deeper into this pose. If you can't see them, try moving your hips back more. Tucking your tailbone under with a microscopic pelvic thrust will keep dat booty from poppin' and protect your lower back.

Transitions: Mountain Pose is the most common transitional pose. Funky alternatives include Twisted Chair Pose, Eagle Pose, or High Lunge.

CHATURANGA

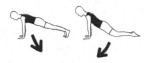
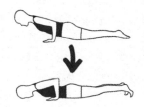

How-To: Start in a Plank Pose. Begin to lower your body reeeaaal slowly. Keep your elbows tight into your body as you go, engaging the hell out of your core and the muscles between your shoulders. Maintain a strong line through your body as you continue lowering, forward and down, until your body is laying on the mat. Once you've landed, your elbows will be tight to your body and pointing upwards. Your hands will be right behind your armpits.

Tips: Use your core and shoulder engagement to keep your shoulder blades from lifting and to prevent your chest from dropping. Keep your neck engaged and in line with the rest of your spine. Also! If coming down from a full Plank Pose is too much, try the same motion starting from your knees in a Half Plank Pose.

Transitions: Chaturanga is a great transition in to Child's Pose or Upward Dog.

CHILD'S POSE

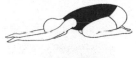
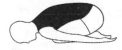

How-To: Kneeling on your mat, bring your tailbone to your heels. While keeping your booty over your heels, walk your hands forward. Let your upper body lengthen, lowering down until your forehead rests on the mat. Once here, chill the fuck out! Relax your back, neck, and hips. You can also experiment by widening your knees to let your torso come between them, or by straightening your arms down to your heels with the palms facing up.

Tips: Keep checking in throughout your body to relax your muscles because they can be sneaky bastards! They like to tense up when we stop paying attention to them.

Transitions: Common transitional poses include Downward Dog, Upward Dog, and Cat-Cow.

CIRCLE DANCE BREATH

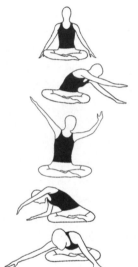

How-To: Begin in a seated position with your legs crossed and inhale both hands overhead. Bring both hands down together and to your right side on the mat. As you exhale, begin drawing a large half circle on the ground with your left hand as it moves across the front of your body on your mat. Your right hand will follow closely behind the other until they reunite on the left side of your body while you finish your exhale. Next, lift your arms up and over with your inhale. Allow them to naturally windmill up then down to the right side of your body. Then begin this circle drawing breath procedure all over again!

Tips: Relax your neck and shoulders as you reach while drawing that half circle. Most importantly, connect to your breath as you move through this one.

Transitions: Seated Flows and Seated Chest Opener compliment this one a whole bunch.

DOWNWARD DOG

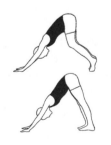

How-To: Begin in a position on all fours. Curl your toes under you and press firmly into your palms as you begin lifting your hips up and back. While your hips rise, straighten your legs as far as is comfortable. Engage from your core down through to your fingertips, aiming to maintain a strong line from your wrists up through to your tailbone. Activate the muscles between your shoulder blades, keeping them in strong alignment by pulling them in and down to your hips.

Tips: Contrary to popular belief, you don't HAVE to straighten your legs all the way or get your heels to the ground in this posture. The line from wrists to tailbone is the key focus here! If this line is hard to achieve comfortably, then try modifying the position of your lower body. You can lift your heels off the mat, bend your legs, or lower your hips.

Transitions: This pose is commonly transitioned into from Mountain Pose or Child's Pose. It's a great lead into many postures! It's especially good for Downward Dog Twists, One-Legged Dog Swings, and Wild Thing Pose.

DOWNWARD DOG TWISTS

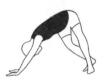

How-To: Get your fine self into Downward Dog. Raise up on your toes and take a slight bend in your knees. Moving them both in the same direction, swivel your knees underneath you and out to the side. Next, swivel both knees underneath you and bring them to the other side. Repeat until that dog feels appropriately twisted.

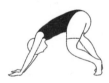

Tips: Remember how important that strong wrist-through-to-tailbone line was in Downward Dog? Yeah? Downward Dog Twists don't give a shit. Allow your hips to raise and lower. Allow your legs to straighten and bend. Let your feet pivot and your body get twisted.

Transitions: Would you be surprised if I said that Downward Dog was a common transitional pose? Alternatively, you can tie together with Foot Stretch or Standing Split.

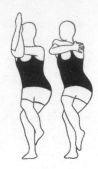

EAGLE POSE

How-To: From standing, shift your weight to begin balancing on one foot. Move your lifted leg overtop the supporting one, crossing at either your ankles or thighs. Next, cross your elbows, then either grab your shoulders or press the backs of your hands together in front of you with your fingertips pointing up. Gently press your elbows up and down into each other. Once your arms and legs are all crossed and such, bend your supporting leg. Keep your core engaged as you lower so that your hips can move backwards as you go.

Tips: Lower backs often default to arching in this pose which can cause booties to pop. This can cause pinching in your lower vertebrae and cause long-term pain. In order to avoid this, keep your lower back straight by engaging your core. Thighs and elbows are crossed and you still feel like you can go farther? Try wrapping your lifted ankle around your supporting calve and/or cross your forearms until your palms are touching.

Transitions: Fabulous transitions include Chair Pose, Standing Leg Swings, and Standing Forward Fold.

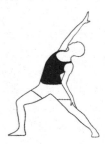

EXALTED WARRIOR

How-To: Begin in Warrior II. Flip your front palm upwards and place your other palm on your back thigh. Engage your core like a freakin' boss, lengthening your spine. Bend at your waist as you come into a side bend, leaning towards your back leg and keeping your chest open toward the side. Lift up and over with your front arm as you lean, reaching farther than dad puns at a holiday dinner. Keep your chest open to the side and lift your gaze.

Tips: Get deeper into this side bend by connecting that badass core power all the way from your legs through to your front fingertips. This will help to lift you as you lean so that you can bend deeper without crunching in on yourself. You can also experiment with your back arm as you get deeper by bending your back elbow and/or positioning your hand farther down your leg.

Transitions: Warrior II is an unsurprisingly common lead-in pose. Warrior II Flows are a great follow up. Try moving through to Airplane Pose if you're feeling real fancy!

FOOT STRETCH

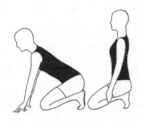

How-To: Get yourself into a tabletop position on all fours. Curl your toes under you so they point forward. Engage your lower abs to lengthen your spine and avoid curving in your lower back. Next, move your hips back to sit on top of your heels. Keep your heels straight up under your butt bones, not flopping out to the side.

Tips: Want to take it easy in this pose? Keep your hands on the ground. Ready for the next level? Rest your hands on your lap (maybe even try out a mudra) and lean back.

Transitions: Foot Stretch is an excellent pose to start off your sequence. It's a great follow up for Seated Flows or Cat-Cow, and it leads well into Child's Pose or Downward Dog.

STANDING FORWARD FOLD

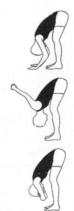

How-To: Stand with your feet about shoulder distance apart. Next, let your upper body melt down, curving your spine forward and letting your arms be heavy. If your knees feel inclined to bend as you melt and fold, then allow them to do so! Once your upper body is comfortably inverted, slowly begin to straighten your legs as far as is comfortable.

Tips: Relax your neck. You can try shifting your weight onto different parts of your foot. Also, relax your neck! Experiment with different arm placements, resting them on the floor or grabbing opposing your elbows. Plus: RELAX YOUR NECK!

Transitions: This pose ties neatly in with Mountain Pose, Standing Back Arch, and Standing Split.

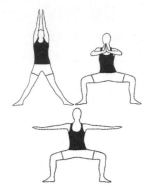

GODDESS FLOWS

How-To: Starting from a Goddess Pose, inhale as you straighten your legs and lift your arms. Bring your hands together to give yourself a high five overhead. As you exhale, bring your hands back down, palms pressed together in "prayer hands." Let your knees bend back into their beginning position in Goddess Pose. On your next inhale, begin this process again.

Tips: Wanna get fancy? Try lifting your gaze up overhead as you give yourself that sweet high five! Make sure that your knees don't collapse inward as you sink back down into Goddess Pose and be sure to keep your spine tall.

Transitions: The main transitional pose is Goddess Pose.

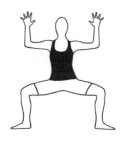

GODDESS POSE

How-To: Start standing with your feet wider than shoulder distance apart and let your feet turn outwards. Engage your core to keep your booty from poppin' as you bend your knees and let your hips sink down, using your quads and booty strength to keep your stance open wide as you go. Continue lowering as far as you comfortably can while maintaining this wide stance. Spread your fingers wide and raise your arms out to your sides in ninety degree angles like those cacti from classic western movies. You know the ones!

Tips: I'm not messing around... Engage your booty and quads! This will keep your knees safe. If your knees absolutely do not like this pose, try sinking less and/or shortening your stance.

Transitions: This pose ties in well with Warrior II, Straitjacket Asana, Wide-Legged Forward Fold, and Extended Side Angle.

GODDESS REACHES

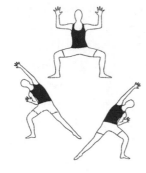

How-To: From a strong Goddess Pose, ground down through one leg and shift your weight onto it as you straighten the other. Bend sideways from your waist toward your supporting leg while reaching your opposite-side arm high, up and over, to get yourself a fan-fucking-tastic side body stretch. Return to Goddess Pose. Repeat process on the other side. Then repeat some more. As you become more comfortable with this motion you can try challenging yourself by lifting your non-supporting foot off the ground as you reach.

Tips: Fast or slow, try to pace these reaches with your breath. You will also get the most out of this pose by making sure that you're not twisting as you lean sideways. Think about your body leaning sideways between two planes of glass so that it can't roll forwards or backwards.

Transitions: The main transitional pose is Goddess Pose.

GODDESS TWISTS

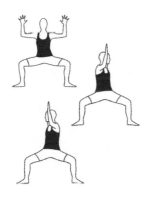

How-To: Begin with a deep inhale in a solid Goddess Pose. Next, exhale as you twist your upper body to one side while maintaining the position of your arms and your lower body. Inhale back to center. Exhale to twist the other way. Inhale to center. Exhale to twist the other way. Repeat.

Tips: Fast or slow, pacing these twists with your breath is key! Keep your legs and booty engaged as you twist in order to stay grounded and keep your hips from tilting or lifting.

Transitions: Number one go-to transitional pose = Goddess Pose!

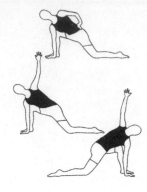

HALF HIGH LUNGE AND TWISTS

How-To: Begin by kneeling on the ground with your hands down on all fours. Next, step one foot forward by your hands. Lift your torso and inhale to bring your hands over-head. Engage your lower abs to scoop your pelvis ever so slightly down and forward. This movement will help you get a fabulous stretch in your back quad and hip flexors while keeping your lower back safe. From here, if it's something you're into, you can progress into Half High Lunge Twists. Return your hands back down to the mat. Raise one arm up toward the ceiling, aiming to create one strong line straight up and down through your arms. If lifting your arm this way is uncomfortable, then rest you hand on your hip instead. Keep your spine long as you enter the twisty portion of this posture, opening your chest to the long side of your mat. Next, you can return your hands back to the mat and raise your other arm to twist the opposite direction.

Tips: Check in with your back leg. Give yourself a stronger foundation by making sure that your shin and the top of your back foot are gently pressing into the ground. When you start to twist in this posture, make sure that whichever hand stays on the mat is beside your front foot. Should it be to the left or the right of your foot? It doesn't really matter! Place your hand on whichever side feels best.

Transitions: Transitions well with Cat-Cow, Warrior I, and Wide-Legged Forward Fold.

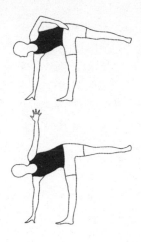

HALF MOON POSE

How-To: Start in a Standing Forward Fold. Walk your hands forward, stacking your shoulders over your wrists and hips over your knees. Engage your core and keep your neck in line with your spine, facing down towards your mat. Lift up onto your fingertips and shift your weight onto one foot. Ease your support onto the hand from the same side of your body as your supporting leg. Ground down through your supporting limbs and power up for the next phase! Raise your non-supporting limbs, opening your arm out to the side and moving your leg straight out behind you. Once steady, slowly open your body to the side to stack your shoulders and hips overtop of themselves.

Tips: Do not forget about engaging and lifting with your non-supporting limbs. Also, this pose can be tricky. If you feel like it's really hard, then it's probably because IT IS! Try modifying with a block under your supporting hand. Try it near a wall. Move slowly. Listen to what your body needs and don't rush it.

Transitions: Standing Forward Fold and Standing Split are most excellent traditional poses.

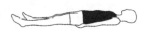

HAPPY ADULT NAP TIME

How-To: Lower your sweet ass self to the mat and lay on your back. Stretch out. Become one with the mat. Welcome to one of the best postures ever. Allow your eyes to close and relax. Allow all the muscles in your face to relax. All them muscles up in your abdomen, arms, and legs? Yeah. They can relax too. Melt into the ground like butter on toast.

Tips: Amplify the benefits of this pose by pairing it with a mediation that best suits you. Make sure you get real comfy too! Try throwing a blanket on top of you if you're cold. You can also get extra snuggly by placing a small roll under your neck or placing a pillow/bolster under your knees. But most importantly: RELAX DAMMIT!

Transitions: Happy Adult Nap Time is key for integrating all the physical and mental benefits of your practice, which is why it is at the end of most Yoga sequences.

HEAD-TO-KNEE POSE

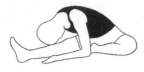

How-To: Bring your fine booty down onto your mat in a seated position. Straighten one leg out in front of you. Bend your other leg out to the side, resting your foot on the inside of your outstretched thigh. Square your hips towards your outstretched leg, pointing both hip bones towards the foot. Engage your core to sit tall and strong! Maintain this posture as you slowly lower your upper body down towards your straightened leg, inching your hands closer to the foot as you go. Once you cannot comfortably lower any farther with this engaged posture, allow your muscles to relax and melt down.

Tips: You can wrap a strap around your foot and use it to pull you deeper into this posture. Or, if you can reach, you can pull on your foot for that extra oomph. Also, despite its name, this pose isn't really about getting your head to touch your knee. It's all about aligning your body properly, lengthening and lowering, breathing and repeating. Oh, one more thing! Relax your fucking neck!

Transitions: This is an excellent follow-up pose for Foot Stretch or Nobody's Puppet. It's also a great lead in for Reclined Figure 4 Pose.

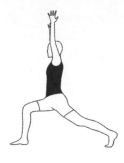

HIGH LUNGE

How-To: From a standing position, shift your weight onto one foot and lift the other. Step your lifted foot far back behind you, planting your toes back on the ground while keeping the heel lifted. Bend your front leg, lining your knee directly overtop your front ankle. Use your core engagement to tuck your tailbone down, scooping your hips ever so slightly underneath you. I like to look at this like the world's tiniest pelvic thrust! Lift your arms overhead. Power up from your legs and pull that strength all the way through to your fingertips. Gaze forward, Badass!

Tips: Watch out for that front knee alignment! Make sure it's stacked right over your ankle by checking if you can see your toes. If you can see the majority of the top of your foot, your knee is too far back. If you can't see your toes, it's too far forward. Ensuring this alignment will save your knees from certain doom (not to be dramatic about it). If your knees already feel like they're in hell, shorten your stance by stepping your back foot in a little closer.

Transitions: Perfect pairing for High Lunge Ski Screams. Also transitions well with One-Legged Dog Swings and One-Legged Mountain.

HIGH LUNGE SKI SCREAMS

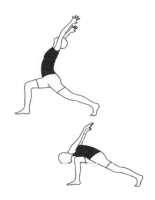

How-To: From a High Lunge, inhale and raise your arms overhead. As you exhale, lean your upper body forward and then lower your chest down towards your front thigh. As you descend, get vocal with your exhale and bring your arms forward and behind you. As the name implies, when you do this you'll look kinda like a screaming skier! On your following inhale bring your breath in through your nose and lift your upper body back into your starting position. Repeat three or more times.

Tips: As you raise and lower your upper body be sure to stay strong and grounded through your lower body. You can modify the speed of your "ski screams" to your liking. You can also modify the height. If screaming in a High Lunge isn't comfortable, you can kneel on your back knee and get your skis on in a Half High Lunge.

Transitions: This ties is smoothly with High Lunge and Half High Lunge. More adventurous transitions include Exalted Warrior and Half Moon Pose.

LET THAT SHIT GO BREATH

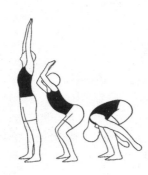

How-To: Inhale and bring your arms overhead in a standing position. Next, let gravity do its thing! Allow your upper body to flop forward, arms and all. As you embrace your floppiest self, use your diaphragm to add extra oomph to your exhale. There are probably going to be some strange noises as this breath is expelled from your mouth. Let that happen. Let it be raw or powerful or awkward. Let it be a whole sentence you've just needed to scream all day, coherent or otherwise! Once you've reached your maximum floppiness and have expelled all your air/noises, roll back up to standing as you inhale back to your starting position. Repeat three or more times.

Tips: If you have low blood pressure or are prone to dizziness, make sure to take your time coming back up to a standing position. In these cases, or if you have an injury that makes flopping uncomfortable, you can do this breath while sitting in a chair.

Transitions: Mountain Pose naturally leads into this breath. Some excellent follow-up postures include Standing Forward Fold or Chair Pose. Or you can melt to the ground after the exhale to transition into seated postures.

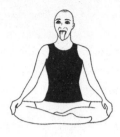

LION'S BREATH

How-To: Begin in a comfortable seated position. Close your eyes. Pull air deep into your belly as you inhale through your nose. Allow the breath to roll up into your chest and expand your rib cage. Next, as you exhale through your mouth, open your eyes as wide as possible and stick your tongue out as far as you humanly can! If your breath makes an airy "haaaaa" sound and you feel as though you look like a mythical fire breathing demon (or Gene Simmons) then you're doing it right. On your next inhale, close your eyes and relax. Repeat this Lion's Breath three more times.

Tips: Relax your face, especially your eyes, on your inhale. On your exhale, your tongue should stick out so far that you feel it stretch. A tongue stretch might sound weird but, just like any other muscle, it's connected to a network of other fun bodily components and it's worthy of some tender loving care too.

Transitions: Although this breath is most commonly done while sitting cross-legged, it can be done in any posture. If you're feeling particularly fierce, try pairing it with Warrior I, Warrior II, or High Lunge.

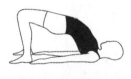

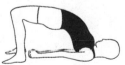

LITTLE BRIDGE

How-To: Start by laying on your back and bending your knees. Extend your fingertips down towards your heels and keep your heels close to dat booty. Ground down through your feet as you raise your hips, doing an awkward and/or sassy pelvic thrust towards the ceiling. Scoot your shoulders closer together underneath you to create extra room to lift and get that chest-opening action going on. You can deepen this pose by interlacing your fingers underneath you to create a strong foundation to push into as you power up your hips.

Tips: Double check to make sure your knees aren't caving in towards each other. You want to keep them aligned over your ankles. Try squeezing your butt muscles and lifting from your hips instead of from your stomach. This will help stretch into your hip flexors instead of your lower back.

Transitions: Ties in well with the likes of Reclined Figure 4 and Reclined Butterfly. Wind Relief Pose is kick-ass follow-up posture.

MOTHER FUCKIN' UNICORN

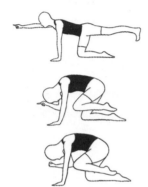

How-To: Begin on all fours, hips stacked over your knees and shoulders over your wrists. On your inhale, extend one arm forward as you extend your opposite side leg straight back while keeping your foot flexed. On your exhale, bring your raised knee and elbow together underneath you as you arch your back and drop your head. Once you're comfortable in this motion, it's time to add some extra majesty! Transform your lifted hand into a fist unicorn by turning up your middle finger. You can transform yourself into a unicorn by touching that middle finger to your forehead before extending it out with your inhale. Repeat three times.

Tips: Some people prefer to extend on the exhale and arch on the inhale. Neither is inherently right or wrong so give them both a try and find which you prefer. Extra tip: aim to keep your extended leg at the same height as your back. And do BOTH SIDES!

Transitions: This is a great follow-up to Cat-Cow. Also pairs nicely with Child's Pose and Piss On Everything.

MOUNTAIN POSE

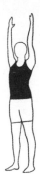

How-To: Mountain Pose is deceiving because it just looks like standing...but it's so much more! Begin with your toes pointing forward, shoulder distance apart. Lift your toes up and put them down one at a time, thinking about getting yourself a firm grip on the mat. Next, take a slight bend in your knees and think about pulling badass energy all the way up from the ground as you straighten them again. This will engage all of the muscles in your legs and power up your core. Follow this engagement into your chest as you inhale your hands overhead. Now you're a super strong mountain that not even the Incredible Hulk could push over!

Tips: The key to any super strong badass mountain is a solid foundation. Focus on your feet and ensure your weight is spread evenly throughout the entire bottom of your foot. You can also think of kicking your heels inwards ever so slightly to give your leg muscles some extra oomph.

Transitions: Mountain Pose can transition to/from damn near everything. For the sake of listing a couple: High Lunge, Standing Leg Swings, Forward Fold, Chair Pose, etc.

NINJA LUNGES

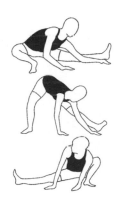

How-To: Start off in a Wide-Legged Forward Fold with your hands on the ground. Next, begin shifting your hips from side to side. Allow your knees to bend and straighten as you start getting experimental. Move your hands around, rise up onto your toes or your heels, try lifting and lowering your hips and torso. The key word here really is "experiment." Explore how your movements change the sensations in your body.

Tips: See if you can find a rhythm that feels really fucking good, and if you can, connect it to your breath. And why not toss some invisible throwing stars while you're at it? Bonus points for sound effects.

Transitions: The most common entrance and exit posture is Wide-Legged Forward fold. Honorable mentions go out to Goddess Pose and High Lunge.

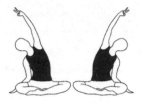

NOBODY'S PUPPET

How-To: While seated on dat fine booty, rest your hands beside you on the mat. Inhale one arm up overhead as you lean towards the other side for a gentle side bend. As that arm reaches up overhead, turn your gaze towards the ceiling and imagine there are strings dangling over you. Now imagine your reaching hand transforming into a pair of badass scissors. Cut those dastardly strings as you exhale, bringing your hand back to the mat before you inhale to repeat this motion on the other side. Repeat three or more times on each side.

Tips: Those strings can represent anything that is holding you back or that you want to free yourself from. Self-doubt, expectations, fear... Whatever it might be, imagine cutting those strings and freeing yourself from its attachment to you. You're a majestic badass, you're nobody's puppet, dammit!

Transitions: Ties in wonderfully with the likes of Seated Flows and Seated Scoop Breaths.

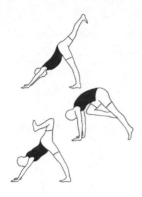

ONE-LEGGED DOG SWINGS

How-To: Begin in a Downward Dog posture. Next, inhale as you lift one leg up high. Keep this lifted leg straight, thinking about sending power all the way up your body, back and up through your leg, then out your foot. Bend your lifted leg on your exhale as you bring your knee in towards your chest. Allow your back to arch and your body to shift forward, taking more weight into your hands as you move through this motion. Repeat this motion, using the lift of your inhale to send your leg back and up, using the force of your exhale to curl and shift forward. Do so three or more times.

Tips: Lower your head as you arch your back to keep your neck in line with your spine. If you want to increase the intensity of these swings, try to shift as much weight as possible back into your legs as you can as you inhale. Then try shifting as much as you can forward into your hands with your exhale.

Transitions: These are a great lead-in for Warrior II, High Lunge, and Wild Thing Pose.

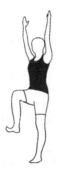

ONE-LEGGED MOUNTAIN

How-To: From a strong Mountain Pose, start shifting your weight onto one foot. Ground down though your support-ing leg and engage your core as you bend your lifted leg into a right angle. Aim to have the thigh of your lifted leg parallel to the ground.

Tips: Pick an unmoving spot to focus on to help you bal-ance. Also, there is no definitive way to hold your hands in this posture. Play around, find your favorites and try out some mudras.

Transitions: You can easily step your lifted leg back into postures like Airplane Pose, Warrior I, or Warrior II.

ONE-LEGGED OPEN MOUNTAIN

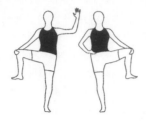

How-To: Begin in a One-Legged Mountain Pose. Next, place the hand from the same side of your body as your lifted leg on the inside thigh of your lifted leg. Press gently into your thigh, slowly opening your leg out to the side, as you stay balanced and rooted down through your supporting leg. Aim to keep your lifted leg in a right angle as it opens up. Bring your other arm out to the side in a right angle with our fingertips pointed towards the ceiling.

Tips: Try engaging the muscles in the side of your butt. This will help your lifted leg move out to the side by opening up your hip.

Transitions: The obvious transitional posture is Mountain Pose. More adventurous transitional postures include Eagle Pose, Chair Pose, and Bob's Cosmic Dancer.

PARTY PEOPLE

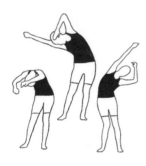

How-To: Start off in a standing position with your arms overhead. Next, exhale and gently lean over to one side. Inhale back up and then exhale over to the other side. Keep doing this then... make it weird! While staying connected to your breath, try bending your knees and dropping your head down as you curl forward. Try bending your elbows and shifting your hips from side to side. Fuck around, find what feels good, then do more of it.

Tips: This posture has been named as such because it often makes you look like you are rocking out, flailing your hands in the air like you just don't care. Embrace that and have yourself a badass party!

Transitions: This ties in nicely with Standing Back Arch, Picking Apples, and Let That Shit Go Breath.

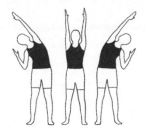

PICKING APPLES

How-To: Bring thy fine self into a standing position with your arms overhead. On your exhale, begin to lean to one side as you lower the elbow from that side down towards your hip. Tilt your head slightly towards this side too, completing the sideways bend in your spine, and reach your other arm up and over. Inhale back to your starting position. Exhale as you repeat this motion to the other side. Repeat this three or more times on each side.

Tips: When you lean to one side, try to ground the foot from the opposite side firmly down into the mat. This will increase the awesomeness of your side stretch and expand it into your hips. Don't miss out on the full stretch by shifting your weight onto one foot!

Transitions: Picking Apples can easily get wacky and transition to Party People. Other transitions include Chair Pose and Standing Back Arch.

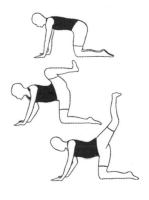

PISS ON EVERYTHING

How-To: Start off on all fours with your hips stacked over your knees and your shoulders over your wrists. Keeping it in a right angle, lift one leg out to the side. Next, begin drawing circles with your raised knee. Start small and slowly let them get bigger. As these circles grow and become more wild, allow your torso to open up to the side and your hips to shift back and forth. You'll know you're doing it right when your hips and back feel groovy and when you look like a dog marking its territory.

Tips: PISS. ON. EVERYTHING.

Transitions: Try pairing this with Child's Pose, Mother Fuckin' Unicorns, or Downward Dog.

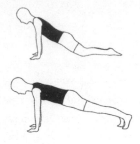

PLANK POSE

How-To: Begin by laying on your stomach, resting your forehead on the mat. Place your hands on the mat by your sides with your fingertips up near your armpits. Keep your arms tight to your body with your elbows pointing up to the ceiling. Engage your shoulder muscles to pull your shoulder blades in and down your back. Fire up your core, curl your toes underneath you, and push into your hands as you straighten your arms. Keep your gaze down to your mat so your neck stays in line with your spine. Don't forget to breathe!

Tips: This pose is often modified by lowering down onto the forearms and/or knees.

Transitions: Common transitions include Downward Dog and Upward Dog.

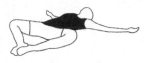

RECLINED BUTTERFLY

How-To: Lay down on your back and bend your knees with your heels together. Open your arms, laying them out to your sides with palms facing up. Let your knees fall away from each other and out to the sides, creating a diamond shape with your legs. The next and most crucial step is just chill out! Relax your stomach as you take steady breaths, allowing your chest and hips to open.

Tips: It's hard to "chill out" if you're uncomfortable. There are many ways you can use pillows or bolsters to support your body for maximum goodness. You can place these under your knees to open your hips or under your shoulders to open your chest. Fuck it! Why not just throw a blanket over yourself and meditate about it? Or take a nap? You've earned it.

Transitions: Sequences well with the likes of Reclined Figure 4, Reclined Twists, and Wind Relief Pose.

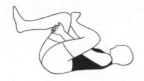

RECLINED FIGURE 4

How-To: Begin by laying on your back. Next, bend your knees and bring your heels towards your booty. Raise one leg, letting your knee fall out to the side and flexing your foot. Place this lifted ankle just above the knee of your other leg, creating a shape that resembles the number 4. Bring the hand from the same side of your body as your lifted leg through the middle of this fancy new leg 4. Bring your other hand into the mix, interlacing your fingers around the back of your thigh or the front of your shin.

Tips: Take extra notice of your hips and shoulders and think about smoothing them into your mat. Keep taking deep breaths, letting your stomach expand. This breath can drastically change how this posture feels and multiply its benefits.

Transitions: A fabulous follow-up posture is Little Bridge. This also ties in nicely with Wind Relief Pose, and Reclined Butterfly.

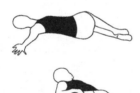

RECLINED TWISTS

How-To: Lay down on your back and bend your legs at a 90° angle as though you are sitting in an invisible chair. Open your arms wide and rest them on the ground. Move your knees together as one unit, closer than two best friends at summer camp, letting them lower to the ground on one side of your body. You can deepen this posture by taking the hand from this side of your body and resting it on your top knee. Next, if comfortable, turn your head to the other side. This will bring the twist up into your neck and get your whole spine involved in this badass twisty goodness.

Tips: Make sure to keep your spine long and ensure all parts of your spine are contributing to the twist. Otherwise you can put too much strain on one area of your back of your back.

Transitions: An awesome follow-up posture is Happy Baby. Reclined Butterfly, Little Bridge, and Wind Relief Pose sequence well too.

SEATED CHEST OPENER

How-To: Begin in a seated position with your legs either crossed or extended straight out. Place your hands behind you on the mat. Engage your shoulders back and down to create space for your chest to open forward and up toward the ceiling. Push onto your hands, engage your core, and keep opening your chest as you bring this active engagement into your neck. Lift your chin up and back.

Tips: You can deepen this pose by taking a microscopic bend in your elbows or by pulling your palms towards the back of your mat while keeping them firmly planted down.

Transitions: Sequences well with Cat-Cow, Seated Scoop Breaths, and Child's Pose.

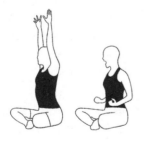

SEATED FISTS OF FIRE

How-To: From a seated position with your legs crossed, inhale as you lift your hands overhead. Next, clench your hands into fists and quickly pull them down to your hips with your wrists facing up and elbows tight to your body. Exhale as you make this motion. Don't half ass this exhale! Let it come out through your mouth, quick and sharp. It might make a deep "hoo" or higher "ha" sound. Or you can get real vocal with it and turn this exhale into a full on battle cry! Repeat this process, inhaling hands overhead and exhaling them down into fists. Repeat this move three or more times.

Tips: Use the power of your exhale to engage your core

and force the air out of you. You can also add extra intensity to this breath by leaning back and lifting your feet off the mat with every exhale.

Transitions: This ties in well with Circle Dance Breath, Piss On Everything, and Downward Dog.

SEATED FLOWS

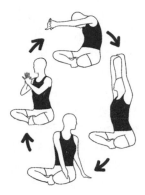

How-To: Begin in a seated position with your legs crossed. Take a badass breath in with your hands in a prayer position in front of your chest. Interlace your fingers as you exhale, pushing your palms forward and arching your back while you lower your head. Keep your fingers interlaced and sit up tall with your next inhale, straightening your arms overhead as though you're pushing the ceiling away. Come into a Seated Spinal Twist with your next exhale, moving one arm down and across your body to your opposite side knee. On your following inhale return back to your starting position, facing forward with your hands in a prayer position. Twist to the other side as you repeat this process. Twisting each way = one repetition. Do three or more repetitions.

Tips: You already know what I'm going to say, right? Connect to your breath! Use your inhales to lift and the force of your exhales to charge up your core and deepen these motions, especially that spinal twist at the end!

Transitions: Seated Flows can be a great start to any sequence. They also pair well with Seated Chest Opener and Seated Forward Fold.

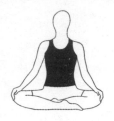

SEATED LEGS CROSSED

How-To: Cross your legs in a seated position. Let's be real, most people have done this since they were children! However, we're going to bring some extra mindfulness into it. From this crossed-legged position, lean back a tiny bit and scoop your pelvis forward under you. This will help lightly engage your core, giving you a solid foundation so you can find the true center point to stack your vertebrae over. Sit tall and allow your shoulders to drop. Rest your hands wherever they feel groovy.

Tips: Grabbing dat butt meat and pulling it out to the sides will help you sit more firmly on your mat. Try to keep your weight even on each of your sitting bones.

Transitions: This can easily transition into any seated posture. It sequences well with anything that begins on all fours such as Piss On Everything or Mother Fuckin' Unicorn.

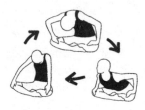

SEATED SCOOP BREATHS

How-To: In Seated Legs Crossed place your hands on top of your knees. Inhale, bending elbows out to the sides and bringing the top of your head down. Continue following this inhale, swooping your torso forward and up as though you just gave your mat a real big sniff. Use your hands to pull yourself forward as lift through your scoop, opening your chest upwards and finishing your inhale. As you exhale, arch your back and lower your head as you straighten your arms. While maintaining this arch, lean aaaaaaaaaaaall the way back until your knees start to lift. Repeat this breath again, scooping with your inhale and arching back with your exhale. Repeat this move 3 or more times.

Tips: As you open up at the top of your inhale you can get a bit of extra stretch into the front of your neck by tilting your chin up. Be careful if you partake in this extra neck extension. Move slowly, lengthening your neck up AND back.

Transitions: Transitions work with Seated Chest Opener, Circle Dance Breath, and Seated Flows.

SEATED SPINAL TWIST

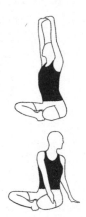

How-To: Begin in a seated position with your legs crossed. Lift your hands overhead and then bring them down and across your body, resting one hand on your opposite side knee. Place your other hand on the mat behind/beside you, wherever it feels right. Keep your spine super tall and long as you press your first hand into your knee to get that twisty goodness. If you feel so inclined, you can bring this twist all the way up into your neck by turning your gaze to look at the wall behind you.

Tips: Make sure that you're keeping your posture super tall as you twist. This length will help you evenly distribute the work to all parts of your back instead of pissing one off by overworking it.

Transitions: This ties in wonderfully with any seated position. Common transitions include Seated Chest Opener, Circle Dance Breath, and Nobody's Puppet.

SIDE ANGLE POSE

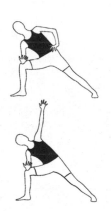

How-To: From a Warrior II Pose engage your core and lengthen your spine. Maintain this strong and lengthened posture as you begin to reach forward with your front arm. Next, rest your front elbow on top of your front knee, turning your forearm upwards so that your open palm faces the ceiling. Aiming to stack your shoulders vertically, raise your back arm up to the ceiling. Engage your booty to help open your hips to the long side of your mat, thinking about your front hip moving toward it and the other rolling away.

If it feels right, allow your back foot to turn out slightly to accommodate this opening rotation.

Tips: Use your raised hand for lift to avoid dumping all of your weight into your front elbow. See if you can feel how this lift can be generated from your legs to your core then all the way through your raised hand. It's fucking magical. PS: if it's uncomfortable overhead, bring your raised hand down to your back hip and think about lifting through your shoulder instead.

Transitions: This is a great lead-in pose for Plank Pose, High Lunge, and Exalted Warrior.

SINGLE LEG LOWERS

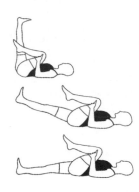

How-To: Begin by laying on your back and hugging your knees tight into your chest. Next, let go of one leg and extend it upwards with your foot flexed. Continue hugging the other knee tight into your body, grabbing either behind your thigh or reaching around to the front of your shin. Keep your torso long and engage your core, flattening your shoulders and lower back to the mat. Think about extending all the way through to the heel of your lifted leg as you begin to lower this leg to the ground. Move slowly, taking your sweet time, and keep this lengthened engagement for a couple breaths once your heels has reached its new home on your mat. Next, pull both knees tight into your body and reset to complete this motion with your other leg.

Tips: As your leg lowers, keep your core strong to help your shoulders and lower back stay on the mat.

Transitions: This is a great lead-in for Wind Relief Pose. It also sequences well with Reclined Twists and Little Bridge.

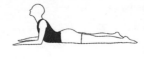

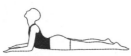

SPHINX POSE

How-To: Lay on your stomach and bring your elbows underneath your shoulders. Spread your fingers wide and plant down firmly through your forearms to give yourself a strong base in your upper body. Exhale as you ground down through your forearms and let your shoulders come down away from your ears. Leave your bottom ribs down on your mat as you inhale, lengthening your spine up to lift through your chest and neck. For extra intensity, focus on expanding your chest with your inhales and gently pulling your palms back towards you with your exhales.

Tips: Sure, most of the cues for this posture are happening in your upper body, but this doesn't meant your lower body gets to go on vacation! Keep your legs lengthened and lightly pressed into your mat.

Transitions: This posture plays nice with Child's Pose and Upward Dog.

STANDING BACK ARCH

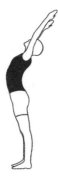

How-To: From a super strong standing position, inhale and bring your arms up overhead. Check in on your feet, making sure you have a strong connection to the mat and feel grounded through your legs. Power up your core and use your next inhale to lift through your chest, bringing your gaze up towards your fingertips. Use the strength of your next exhale to reach up and slightly backwards, staying firmly grounded through your legs. Continue using your breath to lift and support your upper body as it continues arching backwards, slowly deepening this posture.

Tips: Keep your neck in line with your spine. Trying to lift it out of this alignment, or letting it lean back all floppy-like, is an easy way to get hurt. So...don't!

Transitions: Top notch transitional postures include Mountain Pose, Chair Pose, and Standing Forward Fold.

STANDING LEG SWINGS

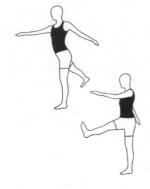

How-To: Start off in a standing position and then shift your weight onto one foot, allowing the other to just barely leave the floor. Next, let this lifted foot begin to sway back and forth. Whenever it feels right, give this sway a little extra energy so that it gets higher and/or faster. Let it start to develop a rhythm of its own as your arms join in on the party, swaying to counterbalance your leg as it goes back and forth.

Tips: Take your time to find the rhythm and connection between your arms and legs as they move. This connection is way more important than swinging your leg super high or super fast! Start slow and steady and move from there.

Transitions: Choice transitional postures include Bob's Cosmic Dancer, Eagle Pose, and Party People.

STANDING SPLIT

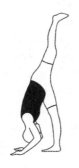

How-To: Begin in a standing position with your body folded forward and your hands on the mat. Shift your weight onto one foot and lift the other up straight behind you with your foot flexed. Keep your neck in line with your spine as your straighten your arms to push your weight back into your hips. Make sure that both of your hip bones are facing towards the mat or towards your supporting leg instead of twisting open to the side. Keep pushing back into your hips as your engage the crap out of your lifted leg, creating a strong line from your wrists through to your raised heel.

Tips: Despite what the name might imply, this pose isn't about doing the splits. Sure, the alignment has the same key components and the same muscles get stretched, but this pose is all about that wrist-through-to-raised-heel connection.

Transitions: This posture plays nice with Half Moon Pose, Warrior I, and Standing Forward Fold.

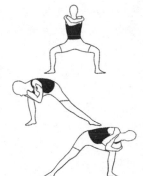

STRAITJACKET ASANA

How-To: Get your divinely Badass Self into a Goddess Pose. Next, open your arms wide and then sweep them across your chest to grab your opposite side shoulders. You'll know you've done it right when you look as though you're giving yourself a big ol' hug and/or as though you're wearing an invisible straitjacket. Start to bend and straighten your legs as you shift your weight from side to side. Keep rocking and get experimental with your posture. Try rocking with varying degrees of intensity. Try letting your torso lower, sway, and twist in whichever ways feel groovy. Try letting your neck get in on the action, gently rolling as you move.

Tips: Wriggle! Writhe! Get weird!

Transitions: Goddess Pose, Wide-Legged Forward Fold, and High Lunge are fabulous transitional postures.

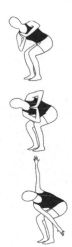

TWISTED CHAIR POSE

How-To: Begin in a Chair Pose with your hands in front of your chest in a prayer position. Next, while keeping your hands in prayer position, lower one elbow down and across your body towards your opposite side knee. Avoid letting dat booty pop by engaging your core and scooping your pelvis forward underneath you. Keep your spine super long and keep going until you reach your maximum depth. Double check to make sure your weight is even between both of your feet and that your knees are stacked right over your ankles. Next, bring this twist all the way up into your neck by turning your gaze out to the side, then up.

Tips: Make sure your twist is coming from all areas of your back instead of dumping the work solely into one spot. If your elbow can reach across to your opposite side knee, you can press them lightly into each other to push just a little deeper into this posture.

Transitions: Sequences nicely with postures such as One-Legged Mountain, Standing Forward Fold, and Airplane Pose.

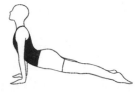

UPWARD DOG

How-To: Begin by laying on your stomach. Place your hands flat on the mat with your fingertips spread wide, keeping your hands and elbows close to your ribs. Engage your shoulders, pulling them in and down your back. Rest your forehead on the mat. Next, press down into your hands as you straighten your arms, slowly lifting your upper body from the ground. Your hips will lift next and, if comfortable, your knees will follow. Lengthen the hell out of your spine and bring your gaze slightly upwards.

Tips: Keep your legs engaged and some pressure into the tops of your feet. This will help you engage your core and scoop your pelvis forward underneath you, which will pro-tect your lower back. A common modification for this pose is to leave your knees on the mat.

Transitions: Try sequencing this with Sphinx Pose, Child's Pose, or Downward Dog.

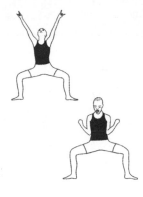

VICTORIOUS GODDESS BREATHS

How-To: Get your divine self up into a Goddess Pose. Next, inhale as you straighten your legs and stretch your arms out wide overhead with your hands in fists. Let your following exhale come out through your mouth, pursing your lips to make an O shape so that your breath creates an audible noise as you force it out. Move with this exhale, bending your knees back to your starting Goddess Pose position and bringing your elbows down into your sides. Repeat! Inhale as your limbs lift and straighten. Exhale loudly as your muscles contract and your limbs bend once again. Do this five or more times.

Tips: As you move though this breath be aware of the engagement in your legs and booty. They are the key to opening your hips and externally rotating from them. This will widen your stance and protect your knees by preventing them from rolling inwards, ensuring that they are pointing in the same direction as your toes.

Transitions: This pairs well with the likes of Wide-Legged Forward Fold and Straitjacket Asana.

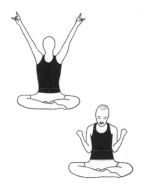

VICTORY BREATHS

How-To: Get yourself into a comfortable seated position. Inhale to lift your arms up wide overhead with your hands clenched into fists. With your following exhale, purse your lips to make an O shape and force your breath sharply out through your mouth. Let this breath be loud as you pull your elbows down tightly into your sides. Repeat! Inhale as you raise your arms overhead. Exhale through your O mouth as you pull your elbows down. Do this five or more times.

Tips: If you wanna, try lifting your chin a tiny bit with your inhales and tucking it with your exhales. If that modification feels good, you can bring your shoulders into the equation by gently pulling them back with your inhales and curling them forward with your exhales.

Transitions: This breath is best friends with Seated Flows and Seated Chest Opener.

WARRIOR I

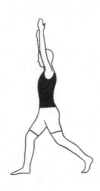

How-To: Start off in a standing position and then step one foot back. Step this foot approximately half the length of your mat. Stay up on your back toes and double check to make sure both of your hip bones are pointing forwards to the top of your mat. Take a slight bend in your back leg and double check to make sure that your front knee is stacked over your ankle. Power up through your legs and into your core as you inhale your arms overhead. Next...breathe. Stay fierce and stay grounded. BOOM!

Tips: Although this is the Warrior I you will see in Rage Yoga, this is a less common approach to the posture. It is more common to see the back foot planted flat and turned out up to about a 45° angle. Your practice is about YOU. Take whichever modification feels right to YOU. The reason Rage Yoga uses the up-on-the-back-toes variation is because the other one can put your knee into a question-able alignment. If your back foot is pointing out but your hip bone is pointing forward, your knee can get caught in the middle and be forced to twist. "Twisty Joints" would be a great '80s post-punk band! However, twisty joints are not always great in your body.

Transitions: Transitioning between High Lunge and Warrior I is easy since the only notable difference is the distance between your feet and the bend in your back leg. Warrior I also plays well with One-Legged Mountain Pose and Warrior II.

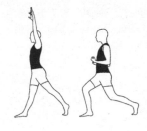

WARRIOR I FISTS OF FIRE

How-To: Begin in a Warrior I position. Inhale, bringing your hands overhead and straightening your legs. Exhale through your mouth, loud and sharp, as you curl your hands into fists and pull them down to your hips. Bend your legs as you move with this exhale, returning them to the same position as they started in Warrior I. Lift with your next inhale as you straighten your legs. As you move with this breath, relax your arms and open your hands as they rise up overhead once again. Repeat! A sharp, loud exhale as you bend your legs and bring your hands into fists is key! Inhale as you straighten your legs and lift your arm. Do this three or more times.

Tips: As you bend your legs with your exhale, watch that your front knee doesn't wander forward past your ankle. Since you're already getting loud with your exhale, why not turn the final one into a full on battle cry? Let that shit go!

Transitions: Chair Pose and One-Legged Mountain Pose are great transitions.

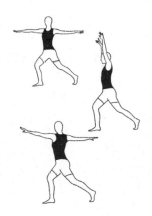

WARRIOR I TWISTS

How-To: Begin in a Warrior I position with your arms raised overhead. Move with your next exhale, twisting your torso and turning your gaze to the open side of your mat. As you twist, bring your arms down to be parallel to the mat, with one reaching forward and the other reaching behind you. Untwist yourself with you next inhale, returning back to Warrior I. Here's where shit gets funky. With your next exhale, bring your arms down again and twist your torso the other direction. You can get your legs involved in the party by straightening them with your inhales and then bending them to their beginning position as you twist with your exhales.

Tips: Does twisting towards the closed side of your mat feel fucked up? Don't worry, you're not alone in this feeling. It helps to keep your spine long to make sure your hips don't turn while you twist.

Transitions: By moving through Warrior I, this sequences well with Standing Back Arch, Eagle Pose, and Chair Pose.

WARRIOR II

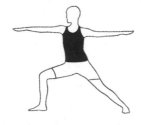

How-To: Get your fine self into a standing position. Lift one leg and step it back about 3/4 of the length of your mat. Allow your back foot to turn out in a 45° angle or until the edge of your foot is parallel to the back of your mat. Bend your front leg to align your front knee directly over your front ankle. Engage your fabulous booty muscles to help your back hip to open and externally rotate your leg. Power up your core as you turn your chest towards the open side of your mat. Bring your arms parallel to the ground with one arm reaching forward and the other reaching back. Turn your gaze forward to look over your fingertips. You can add some extra flavor to this pose by moving your hands into karana mudra or by throwing up a middle finger.

Tips: The external rotation of your back leg is important! This rotation lets your hip bone point open towards the side, which means it can mirror the angle your back foot has turned to. This alignment means your poor knee won't be forced to twist in directions it wasn't designed for. A quick way to see if your front knee is stacked over your ankle is to make sure that you can juuuuuuust see the big toe past your knee.

Transitions: This posture is best friends with the likes of Exalted Warrior, Goddess Pose, and High Lunge.

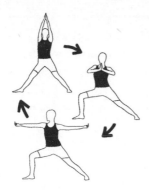

WARRIOR II FLOWS

How-To: Begin in Warrior II. Next, inhale as you straighten your legs and raise your arms directly overhead to give yourself a high five. You deserve it! Breathe out through your nose with your exhale, making some extra noise with your Ujjayi Breath by pressing your tongue to the roof of your mouth. Move with this exhale, bringing your palms together and lowering them down into a prayer position in the middle of your chest. While this is happening, bend your legs back into their starting position. On your following inhale, extend your arms out into their starting position, then lift them overhead as you straighten your legs. Give yourself another big ol' high five and continue the cycling through this flow three or more times.

Tips: Make sure that your front knee doesn't float too far forward as you bend your legs while returning to Warrior II. You can also bring your neck into the flow by keeping your gaze locked on your front fingertips as you move.

Transitions: Aside from the obvious Warrior II transition, this flow ties in well with Exalted Warrior, Goddess Pose, and Warrior I Twists.

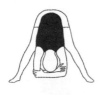

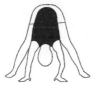

WIDE-LEGGED FORWARD FOLD

How-To: Begin in a standing position. Step your legs wide, taking a badass power stance. Next, hinge at your hips and bend forward. Bring your hands towards the mat and allow your torso to hang heavy. Relax your neck. Ground down through your legs, trusting them to do the work so your upper body can chill to the max. If you feel experimental, try out different arm positions. Try hooking your pointer and middle fingers around your big toes or grabbing your opposite side elbows. You can also interlace your fingers behind your back, then straighten your arms. While you're at it, try swinging your upper body side to side or back and forth.

Tips: Let your feet turn out a little in this wide stance. If you force them to point forward, you can end up putting your knees and ankles into not-so-groovy positions.

Transitions: This posture pairs well with Goddess Pose, Half High Lunge, and Ninja Lunges.

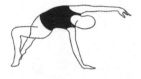
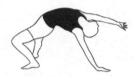

WILD THING POSE

How-To: Start yourself off in a Downward Dog. Lift up onto your toes and begin shifting your weight onto one hand and foot from the same side of your body. Slowly move your non-supporting foot back and then across your mat. As this foot goes about its journey, let your knees bend and lift your hips as they begin to open up towards the side of your mat. As your hips begin this opening rotation, allow your non-supporting hand to lift off your mat, sweeping up overhead as your chest and shoulders open towards the ceiling. Lift your hips up towards the ceiling as well. Keep reaching your lifted arm as you straighten your opposite-side leg to create one solid line of engagement.

Tips: Move slowly and make friends with that cross-body connection because that's what this pose is all about. Bonus: you can do this posture on your knees instead of being all the way up on your toes, and it feels just as fan-fucking-tastic!

Transitions: Top tier transitional poses include One-Legged Dog Swing, Piss On Everything, and Child's Pose.

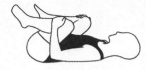

WIND RELIEF POSE

How-To: Sit dat ass down on your mat, then lay on your back. Next, bend your legs and bring your knees towards your chest. Grab behind your thighs or reach around to the front of your knees and hug them in tight. Lengthen your spine with your exhale, flattening your lower back and shoulders to the mat. Take your inhales deep into your belly, feeling your stomach press into your legs and as it expands with your breath.

Tips: Let. Your. Stomach. Expand! We often hold them in so it might feel weird, but this full belly inhale is key here. Relax and focus on the massage-like sensation of your breath as it comes in and out.

Transitions: This posture ties in well with Reclined Twists, Little Bridge, and Happy Adult Nap Time.

ACKNOWLEDGMENTS

Allison Heather-Sides, Drew Stremick, Erin Crossman, and Jinelle Watson. Y'all were the regular crew that made those first classes possible. Thank you so much for your support!

Ang Peters. Sure, you gave me dog food when we were kids, but you also gave me an introduction to rebellion and whimsy! It means a lot to me to have your art in this book.

Chang Lǎoshī. In one of the most grueling times of my life, you always met me with kindness. You taught me that I could stay in one piece when everything falls away.

Chris and Ambor Hewitt. Dickens Pub is where this whole thing took off! Thank you for taking a chance on me. PS: I'm still jealous of your Elvis wedding.

Erin, my slanted sister! You took me on an adventure that opened up my mind in ways I didn't know I needed. I learned so much from your friendship.

Heather Istace. Through the highs and lows, you and Fluffy the Guard Dog have been there. You've been an unwavering support, and I love you.

Josh Dillon. I don't know if we could have had better timing. Thank you for reminding me how to use my voice, to advocate for myself, and that I am exactly enough.

Marion "Mugs" McConnell. Your influence kept my focus lifted. Thank you for readily sharing your wealth of experience and knowledge. You taught me a lot!

The Pat. Accept no imitations, this is THE Pat! You know what you did, you wonderful bitch.

ABOUT THE AUTHOR

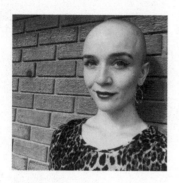 Lindsay Istace is a perfectly normal human worm baby living in Edmonton, Alberta, without any cats. Their career in the world of circus arts (specifically contortion) has lead them to train around the world and is what eventually brought them to yoga. They founded Rage Yoga in 2015. Since then they have continued to work as an artist and yoga instructor. Despite being Canadian, Lindsay does not skate or watch hockey and has never ridden a moose.